A SPECIAL DAY

A SPECIAL DAY

A Mother's Memoir of Love, Loss, and Acceptance After the Death of Her Daughter

ANNE-DAUPHINE JULLIAND

Translated by Adriana Hunter

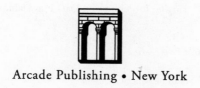

Arcade Publishing • New York

First United States printing 2015 by Arcade Publishing

Originally published in France as Une journée particulière

Arcade Publishing books may be purchased in bulk at special discounts for sales promotion, corporate gifts, fund-raising, or educational purposes. Special editions can also be created to specifications. For details, contact the Special Sales Department, Arcade Publishing, 307 West 36th Street, 11th Floor, New York, NY 10018 or arcade@skyhorsepublishing.com.

Visit our website at www.arcadepub.com.

10 9 8 7 6 5 4 3 2 1

Library of Congress Cataloging-in-Publication Data is available on file.

ISBN: 978-1-62872-449-3
Ebook ISBN: 978-1-62872-477-6

Printed in the United States of America

To Loïc

THE DECIBEL LEVEL OF MY ALARM GOES UP A NOTCH. IT'S insistent now. It must have been going for several minutes, trying to drag me from the depths of a night weighed down by a thousand dreams. I wish I could sleep through 'til tomorrow, buried beneath my comforter. I stretch and reach my hand into the crumpled sheets next to me, but the space is empty and cold—Loïc is up already. I listen intently and make out the sound of the shower.

A jumble of letters and figures spools through my head behind my still closed eyelids. My sleepy mind swirls them around each other before eventually arranging them into a logical order. A date emerges: February 29. Reality takes shape. It's February 29. Today is Thaïs's birthday. My daughter would be eight years old.

Eight already—it doesn't seem possible. What does an eight-year-old do on her birthday? Does she jump out of bed singing? Does she dress up like a princess to mark the day? Does she invite her friends over to blow out her candles? I won't be seeing any of that today. Thaïs's life came to an end more than four years ago. Four and a quarter years, to be precise. The proportions have been subtly inverted: the time she has spent in heaven is now longer than her years with us. Thaïs lived for three and three-quarters years. A short life that totally changed mine.

Her photo always lives on my bedside table. I see her every morning, sitting on the grass with her fuchsia-colored dress fanned out around her, and holding a cookie in her dimpled hand. She's smiling right at the camera, her eyes sparkling. I study her, full of emotion, then my gaze shifts to the book sitting beside the photo frame. I know every detail of its cover, the beach at low tide, the clear sky, the little girl walking with her head turned to look at the ground, her arms stretched out for balance, her bare feet on the wet sand. I pick up the book without opening it, and hold it to me. I know every sentence by heart. They tell the story of Thaïs as told by me. And as lived by me.

I thought my life had been robbed of happiness forever that December night just before Christmas when I felt Thaïs exhale her last breath. I don't need to delve very far into my memory to recall those grim, dark hours. I don't need to dig very deep into my heart to relive the pain. The memories are there, just beneath the surface. A shadow fell across my eyes the moment she left, and I was afraid that I would live in a world deprived of light from then on. I thought I would never experience joy again. Who could still believe in happiness when their child has died? And yet . . .

I spent many years happily ticking boxes. Pretty little square boxes with nice, clear outlines. I didn't have to draw up a list; I instinctively knew what would be on that list—it's dictated by the collective subconscious. So, I had a clear idea of what I needed to be happy. As life went by, I checked off entries like drawing a line through items on a shopping list: "done that." In the space of thirty-two years I'd checked most of the boxes. I was just about to embark on the supplementary list, the one for really lucky people . . . when I came to realize how vacuous the process was.

I had no trouble accepting the first part about childhood and my teenage years: I grew up in a flourishing, loving, united family. I got along well with my brothers and sisters, and loved my parents. My time at school went by practically without a hitch. After graduating high school I embarked on the course I'd wanted to follow for a long time, studying to be a journalist. My transition to adulthood went smoothly. Once I had my diploma, I found a job at a newspaper. Then I met Loïc, the love of my life. We got married, we had a son, and then a daughter—a pigeon pair. We bought an apartment and a car.

We both had jobs that guaranteed us personal fulfillment and a degree of recognition. That's a rough outline of thirty-two years of happiness: happy childhood, check; well-balanced adolescence, check; successful studies, check; interesting job, check; husband and perfect children, check; apartment, car, holidays, check. Life of bliss, check! How great, how wonderful, how perfect.

In all these lists of the codes that make up happiness, there is no place for sickness, pain, and suffering, not even in the margins. So where did my daughter's unusual way of walking fit into all this? Because, at the grand old age of eighteen months, Thaïs didn't have an entirely normal gait. Her feet tilted outward slightly as they touched the ground. I noticed it one late summer's day when I saw her footprints in the wet sand on a beach in Brittany. Loïc and I were just smugly counting all those ticked boxes and contemplating having a third child to ice the cake of our lovely family. I watched Thaïs walk toward me, and looked along the line of footprints she'd left in the sand, thinking I'd feel a surge of maternal pride. I noticed that a bulge of sand had formed on the outside of each footprint. And I didn't like it. Even before anxiety set in, I instantly hated that flawed walk. I saw it as the grain of sand that would jam the cogs of our unimpeachable happiness. I wanted Thaïs to keep her promise of perfection, not to hobble like that. Those awkward little footsteps threw a pebble into our idyllic pond, and went on to whip up a terrible storm.

Sometimes it takes only a moment, just one word to turn a life upside down. The word: "leukodystrophy." The moment: when we were told. Our peaceful existence was blown apart the day Thaïs turned two. Sheltered from prying eyes, in a consulting room at the end of a long corridor in a neuropediatric unit, doctors told us that our daughter had a degenerative neurological condition called metachromatic leukodystrophy. Too many unpronounceable words in one sentence. Her life expectancy would be short and her existence painful. Over the coming months Thaïs would gradually lose all her faculties: the ability to walk, and to move at all, but also the power of speech, her sight, her hearing . . . then she would lose her life. And the last sentence was the cruelest: there is no cure, no form of treatment. No hope. The end of happiness. Or at least of the concept I'd had of it until then.

THE PHOSPHORESCENT NUMBERS ON THE ALARM CLOCK BRING ME back to the present. It's definitely time I get up if I don't want the whole household to be late. I wistfully climb out of the warm covers, slip on a robe, and walk out of the bedroom. A crack of yellow light filters under Gaspard's door. I go in and, among a scrambled-up comforter, I spy a thick mop of hair, a hand gripping an open book, and, behind dark-rimmed glasses, two big brown eyes speeding over the words. Gaspard's already reading at this time in the morning. I tilt my head to make out the title on the cover. Having devoured the whole "Petit Nicolas" series of children's books, Gaspard is now chomping his way through spy novels.

I rumple his hair and tell him it's time to get up. He heaves a sigh.

"Already? I'm on a real cliffhanger."

"Yes, already and quickly. You're going to be late for school."

I always get the same refrain, and it makes me smile every morning. I like his daily protests because it's so fitting for a ten-year-old. For any ten-year-old. I've often worried that Gaspard would grow up too quickly over these ten years. Our family circumstances mean that he was confronted with sickness, suffering, and death at a young age. His image of life has been altered. But he's still developing like most boys his age. He doesn't like school or girls—at least not for now. He'd rather be playing with his friends or letting off steam on the rugby pitch. The difficulties of life haven't robbed Gaspard of his childhood. He's lived it to the full, although he now feels he's turned a corner: on his tenth birthday, he announced that he would now be a preteen until he was thirteen. From then until he was eighteen he'd be experiencing "teen-age angst." There we are, the schedule is all set out. We know what to expect over the next few years. Like any mother, I'm not relishing being confronted with a son in full-blown adolescence, but I'm happy to see that Gaspard is planning on going through these natural stages. It means he's well balanced.

When he's dressed, Gaspard comes to join me in the kitchen. Loïc comes in next, also ready to face the day. We each sit down at our places. My men aren't very talkative at breakfast time. Gaspard helps himself to some orange juice and pours cold milk over his cereal, then disappears behind the cardboard packaging, absorbed in the game that this particular brand prints on the back. Loïc stirs his coffee without a word. Then he breaks the silence, which until then was interrupted only by chocolate-coated cornflakes crunching between Gaspard's teeth.

"Gaspard, do you know what today is?"

"A school day, like all the rest," he replies glibly.

"Yes, but it's February 29. That's a special date."

"I know; it only happens every four years. Actually, I don't think it's fair we have school today. This should be a holiday. I can't see why they give us an extra day at school like that."

"What really matters," Loïc persists, "is today is Thaïs's birthday."

"Oh yes, it is . . . how old would she be?"

"Eight. A big girl, wouldn't you say?"

Gaspard's spoon hovers midway between his bowl and his mouth. His eyes blur into the middle distance as he analyzes the information. He doesn't have an eight-year-old sister. He tries to imagine it, to project himself into a hypothetical present. The spoon continues on its way, and Gaspard speaks through his mouthful: "Do you remember Thaïs well, Mommy? I feel like I'm forgetting her face. Do you get that, too?"

"Yes, sweetheart, I get that a lot. Memories fade with time, but feelings stay the same."

This all seems clear to me now, but I would never dare tell him how terribly I've struggled against the natural failings of the human memory. Yes, you can even forget what you thought was unforgettable. Even your own child's features, the smell of her hair, the feel of her skin. You forget, and there's nothing you can do about it. I felt such panic the first time I asked myself, "Actually, what *were* her eyes like, and her voice, and the warmth of her body?" I felt guilty. I felt I had to do everything in my power to stop time from obscuring my memory with its opaque veils, until I realized that Thaïs was fading in my mind's eye, but not in my heart. The heart's memory is our feelings, and it doesn't suffer any erosion with the passage of time. It is fresh, timeless, unchanging. When I call on my heart's memory, I can conjure impressions inscribed in the very depths of my being. The feelings I had with Thaïs and for her come back to me intact. And I can savor magical moments in which my memory faithfully restores the way Thaïs smelt, the twinkle in her dark eyes, the depth of her sigh. I cry like a baby every time my feelings bring my memories back to life.

"Time to go!" Loïc announces. He's dropping Gaspard at school this morning on his way to work. He takes me gently in his arms and whispers, "I hope you're going to be okay today, my darling. I'll be thinking of you, and her. Eight years ago we brought a wonderful little girl into the world." I cling to him, burying my head in the crook of his neck, dampening his collar with my tears. Yes, a wonderful little girl . . .

Gaspard slips out to brush his teeth and wash his face and hands, puts on his coat, heaves his heavy satchel onto his back, and leaves the apartment with a "Have a nice day, Mommy. See you later." I rush over and jam my foot in the door just before it slams shut.

"Wait, Gaspard; you didn't give me a kiss."

"Mom!" he sighs sulkily. "I'm ten years old. I'm not going to kiss you every time I go out. Kisses are for babies."

My boy wants to be all grown-up already. Still, he doesn't pull away when I plant a long, noisy kiss on each of his cheeks. I hold him to me for a moment before giving him back his freedom. I too wish this could be a holiday, so that we could stay together as a family today.

I step back into the now-silent apartment. Everything feels strangely still. I take refuge under the shower and let the hot water stream over my shoulders for a long time, hoping that I can finally release this recalcitrant muscular tension. Then I wrap myself in a thick towel and leave the steamy bathroom. In my bedroom I stand in front of the open wardrobe, gazing in bewilderment at my carefully folded clothes.

"I don't have anything to wear," I say with a sigh.

This might seem like an incongruous comment to anyone looking at the dizzying piles of clothes in my closet. But I really mean it. I have more clothes than I need, but I don't have anything to wear today, because I can't see what sort of outfit would suit my mood. That's right—my moods have their own sartorial codes; the way I dress depends on how I feel that day. Today nothing in my wardrobe seems to reflect my state of mind. My mood is shaky. Ever since first light it's been hovering between happiness and pain. And it will stay like that 'til after dark.

I knew, even before Thaïs died, that her birthday would be more painful to get through than the anniversary of her death. Of course, memories of the day she died and, even more so, of her funeral are always with me. I can picture that overcast Brittany sky, the hostile darkness feebly illuminated by flickering torches. I can feel the drizzly December chill seeping through our clothes so that our bodies are wrapped in a straightjacket of ice. I see myself kneeling in the cloying wet mud at one end of the gaping hole that will swallow up a part of my very flesh, reeling drunkenly from my tears and the cup of sorrow I've drunk. It's always an ordeal remembering that time.

Memories of Thaïs's birth are perhaps crueler still when you see them through the prism of the rest of her life. I always dreamed of having a daughter. Thaïs's arrival was all I could have wished for. That tiny little baby represented so much promise of happiness to my mother's heart. I now feel contradictory emotions when I remember that day. Every year, between February 28 and March 1, I cry and smile at the same time. I cry for the broken dreams and that terrible absence, and I smile to think of the time I spent with Thaïs. Obviously I wish she could have been healthy, and could live many long years to come, but I don't regret a minute we shared together, those heart-to-heart moments, that precious lifespan. And I'm grateful when I remember everything my daughter taught me. The minute I held Thaïs in my arms for the first time, I felt that I knew I had an ally for life. Not for my life, no; for her life, her three-and-three-quarters-year life. And beyond that, too, because Thaïs is still a precious ally to me.

I decide to leave it to chance. I close my eyes and rummage blindly through the piles of clothes. My hands settle for textures rather than shapes. They plump for a very simple silk top and a comfortingly soft sweater. I open my eyes; chance did a good job: the sweater is purple— Thaïs's favorite color. I complete the outfit with a pair of jeans, high-heeled boots, and matching earrings. Now I'm finally ready to get through today!

I've only just finished getting dressed when a voice calls from behind me. I can hear his little footsteps sliding over the wooden floor; I can smell his sleepy-child smell. From the lilt in his voice, I can tell that his face is lit up with a smile. I crouch down and draw him to me, wrapping my arms around him as tightly as I love him. My little treasure . . .

"GOOD MORNING, MOMMY."

"Good morning, my little Arthur. You slept well. It's late, you know."

"I slept well," he agrees, "but I had a 'fog.'"

"A fog? What's that?"

"It's a horrible dream with monsters and wolves. Do you want me to tell you about it?"

"Of course I do. You tell me about your fog."

Arthur launches into one of those breathtaking accounts that he alone has mastered. I can tell by the way his eyes dart around that he's embellishing things as he goes along. The story is a total jumble, but it bristles with terrifying creatures. When he stops, he's almost out of breath from this endless tirade.

"You see what I mean? Scary, huh?"

"Yes, very. Much more frightening than a nightmare."

"What's a nightmare?" he asks.

"It's like a fog . . ."

"Like a 'ninemare' then?"

"Very nearly like a 'ninemare.'"

I'm weak. I can't bring myself to correct his mispronunciations, his "tooshpaste" and "radigator" and "soap duds," all the words he gets wrong, distorts, or appropriates in his own original way. All the words that remind me that my little boy is three and a quarter, that he can walk and talk and is in perfect health. That he's my obsession. Yes, Arthur is my greatest obsession.

Sometimes it's good to love to distraction. To lose your mind over someone, but not your head, just putting aside rational thoughts and listening only to your heart. Loïc and I had been tormented by a longing for another child for some time. We weren't trying to replace Thaïs—the irreplaceable Thaïs! We just wanted to have a baby, like any other couple, that was all. It was a longing that drained me and saddened me because I thought it couldn't be fulfilled. Metachromatic leukodystrophy is inscribed in our genes. We could pass it on to any child of ours from the moment of conception. The terror of suffering all over again locked down my womb; I didn't feel that I could possibly carry another baby. I was terrified and unhappy. One morning Loïc managed to find the words to break down the prison of my fears.

"Okay," he said. "What if we tried to look at the situation differently. Do you feel you could love another child? Do you think you could love that child just as it is, and you could do everything in your power to make it happy?"

"Yes!" I almost shouted. "Yes, I could. That's all I want. To love a baby and make it happy."

"Well, what are we afraid of, then?"

Nine months later, almost a year to the day since Thaïs died, Arthur was born, in perfect health. We overcame our fears; we took a chance on life. Our families congratulated us, welcoming the news with touching enthusiasm. On the other hand, others, some of them close to us, couldn't understand our decision. When people asked us, "But how could you have another baby?" we replied simply, "The way most people do, in private!" This answer wasn't meant to be just a humorous riposte; it really was the truth. The decision to have a baby belongs to us. It is integral to our relationship. It is in no way open to public debate or a referendum. We will never justify our choice to have Arthur to anyone. We can't even explain it. It's a sort of madness, a wonderful madness, the madness of love. And, to quote Blaise Pascale, "the heart has its reasons, of which reason knows nothing."

"I'M HUNGRY, MOMMY. CAN I HAVE MY BREAKFAST?"

Arthur's morning appetite interrupts my thoughts.

"Of course you can. Come on then; I'll get you your breakfast."

I sit him at the table and put a steaming mug of hot chocolate in front of him, along with a glass of orange juice and two slices of bread with a thick coating of chocolate spread. He grabs the bottle of milk, the carton of orange juice, the pot of Nutella, and the box of cereal, and arranges them in a rampart around his place setting, as he does every morning. In between hearty mouthfuls of bread, he carries on describing his dream in even more outlandish detail.

"Good morning, Anne-Dauphine. Good morning, Arthur."

Thérèse has arrived. I didn't hear her key in the lock, or the front door opening and closing. I go out to greet her, and, as she kisses me, she gives me an extra little squeeze of her arms and pats my back.

"You okay?"

"Yes, I'm fine. How about you?"

"Yes. I'll be okay."

For more than five years now Thérèse has been coming in through our front door every weekday. She comes to look after the children. Officially, that's the sum total of her responsibilities, but in practice

Thérèse does much more than that. She takes care of each and every one of us. She landed in our family mid-heartbreak, after we'd been told about Thaïs's illness. We welcomed her as an angel sent from heaven, and she now ensures that our family stays on an even keel. Just having her here has saved us so many times when we were out of our depth. She ran the household when I just couldn't manage it; she looked after Gaspard when I was by Thaïs's bedside. And she did it without ever losing her patience, her smile, or her serenity. Her innate peacefulness is a soothing balm to our souls.

Arthur runs over and leans against her legs, reaching up to her for his morning kisses. He wraps his arms around her neck and presses his mouth to her cheeks.

"Good morning, Dada."

When they were tiny and could say only a few basic words, the children started calling Thérèse "Dada." It's a nickname that stuck. It's their way of giving her an official and very personal position, because Thérèse is like a member of the family—at least she is in each of our hearts. In our heads we all understand that Thérèse has a life away from us, her own weekends, her holidays, her independence. We know that she comes here because this is her job. We also know that she'll leave one day. That freedom gives our relationship the balance it needs.

During an interview I was once asked who in the world I wished I was like. Of course, I'd love to have Elizabeth Taylor's eyes, Julia Roberts's smile, Cameron Diaz's legs, Heidi Klum's figure, Audrey Hepburn's grace, Marie Curie's intelligence, and Camille Claudel's artistic talent. Of course. But not one of those women is a role model for me. Which is why I replied without a moment's hesitation: Thérèse. I wish I could be like Thérèse. For her straightforwardness, her discretion, her good nature, her dependability, her capacity to love, her care of others, her willingness to make connections, and her conscientiousness in doing everything well. I admire all her qualities as well as that special way she has of loving what she's doing rather than doing what she loves.

Thérèse takes Arthur's hand and walks him over to finish his break-fast. She too is now treated to a description of his "fog," in yet another version. While I make a cup of coffee, I explain to Thérèse that I won't be working today—the privileges of a special day. Arthur won't be going to school, either. He's only just recovered from a hefty bout of seasonal flu. Judging by the look of him, he's absolutely fine, but he's only in the first year of nursery school: one day off won't jeopardize his future. It may just be an excuse for me to keep him at home, like a she-wolf who doesn't want her cubs to stray too far. Particularly on a day like today.

"What about Azylis?" Thérèse asks, buttering a slice of bread. "Is she up?"

"No, not yet. She's catching up on sleep. She was tired yesterday evening. I'll go and see if everything's okay."

I walk out of the kitchen and across the apartment to her bedroom. I stop, put my ear up to the door, and listen. Not a sound. I turn the handle softly and tiptoe into the room. Light from the corridor gently eases the room out of darkness, creating subtle shadows. I can make out my daughter in this play of light. I go over to her and see that her eyes are wide open, her mouth already smiling, her little teeth gleaming white. Azylis is awake. She stretches as far as she can, and it's only then that I realize how much she's grown. Her bed will soon be too small for her. I open her hands, uncurl her fingers, and interlock them with my own.

"Hello, princess. I'm happy to see you."

She replies with that gentle smile of hers. I lift her up into my arms, delighted to feel that she's gained weight again.

In four months' time, to the day, Azylis will be six years old. Six—how wonderful to have a daughter who's nearly six. I can already picture her eyes sparkling at the sight of beribboned presents, her dazzling smile as she listens to us singing, her face lit up by the candles on her chocolate cake—that's her favorite. I can see her cheeks filling to blow out the flickering flames. And I know even now that she won't be able to blow them out. I also know that this inability won't spoil her fun, nor ours. On June 29 Azylis won't blow her candles out by herself. On the morning of her birthday we'll draw straws to see which one of us gets to help her. The boys will probably squabble over the privilege. I'll cross my fingers behind my back in the hopes that it will be me. I love celebrating Azylis's birthdays and watching the number of candles go up every year. I'm so terrified that it won't happen.

Azylis was barely a week old when we were told that she was ill. One tiny little week of life, too few days to understand. We were still reeling from the shock of hearing that Thaïs was ill, already busy dealing with new symptoms. Azylis was born in the midst of that torture. Her birth was like a bright spell in the middle of a storm, a brief truce on the battlefield, a precious moment when time stood still. It took a few short days for the doctors to do their tests, check the results, and tell us that our baby was also suffering from meta-chromatic leukodystrophy.

Do I really have to relive that shock? Do I need to remember the words spoken, the silences? Do I have to go back over the pain, fear, and darkness of that day? There are words to describe what we felt, but I have no desire to summon them. I'll keep them buried deep inside me, like a secret. And it is probably the most intimate kind of secret, because it is the secret of fear.

Thérèse comes into the room behind me, and Azylis smiles a little more widely as Thérèse approaches. The complicity between them is quite unique. They know each other and understand each other perfectly. They came into our family at almost the same time. Thérèse was in close attendance for Azylis's birth, the news that she was ill, and what followed. What followed was something quite unexpected, a mad adventure we threw ourselves into: a bone marrow transplant for Azylis. On the strength of her bad test results, the doctors who were dealing with us, and who were specialists in leukodystrophy, mentioned this option. A bone marrow transplant was our only hope, giving us the tiniest chance of curing our baby. At her very young age she didn't yet show any obvious signs of the illness, no out-turned feet, no shaking hands, no stammered words. We had the time to try something, time we didn't have in Thaïs's case. We agreed, without knowing where this experiment would take us.

In the first instance, it took us from Paris to Marseille, to the transplant facility of a major local hospital. Without the slightest hesitation, Thérèse left everything behind to come with us. She moved in with us and stayed for the duration of our momentous time in Marseille—four long months. She shared our hopes and fears. She shared our tears and triumphs. And still does to this day.

THE BATH IS READY. THÉRÈSE HAS RUN THE WATER AT THE PERFECT temperature, poured in the sweet-smelling oil, and set up the sling in the bottom of the tub. Azylis is quivering with impatience as Thérèse lays her down in it. My little girl wouldn't miss her morning bath for anything in the world. It gives her a good start to the day and dispels the stiffness of a night of immobility. Water frees her from her own weight; her arms and legs can stretch out and become more supple. Azylis savors this moment of relaxation. Thérèse, Arthur, and I are there to share in her pleasure, the three of us gathered around the bathtub as courtiers would once have done for a king.

Azylis has not been cured. She probably never will be. But we believed she was long after her treatment was over. Right up until her little foot started lagging behind. Right up until her walk slowed down. Right up until we faced the facts: Azylis is still sick.

Deep inside me, the words of the academic and emeritus oncologist professor Jean Bernard still resonate: "Add life to the days when you can't add days to the life." Those words saved us when we were told that Thaïs was sick. They set us back on track, showing us which path to follow: the path of everyday life, of the moment, of doing things. A day

as a whole lifetime. Professor Bernard's words are still significant
now. The transplant meant that we could add days to Azylis's life; it
changed the course of her life. But it didn't save it. When she was
eighteen months old, Azylis was lively, alert, and flourishing. No
one would have suspected what she'd endured in her first year. She
showed no aftereffects, except perhaps for a lack of appetite and
slightly low bodyweight. Nothing serious. I watched out for her first
steps avidly, looking out for the slightest sign of the illness. One
day she took the plunge . . . and walked perfectly normally. And I
stopped my anxious trembling.

Then her foot started turning outward. And I stopped believing in
the cure.

Before all this, I knew nothing about metachromatic leukodystrophy.
I didn't know a single fact about its pathology, or even that it existed at
all. Doctors explained this "incurable, degenerative, genetic, neurologic
disorder" to us: a missing enzyme. Just one, one tiny enzyme, and it too
had the most unlikely name, but without it the whole beautiful machin-
ery of a human body seizes up and breaks down. Without this enzyme,
the myelin sheath that surrounds our nerves gradually disintegrates,
like taking the casing off an electric cable. And without myelin, nerves
can no longer transmit information from the brain to the muscles. The
problem first affects motivity before moving on to vital functions.

Unfortunately, I now know a lot about this condition. I lived through
it with Thaïs. I watched her abilities and her senses dwindle. I dreaded
each stage and each decline. I knew what would happen. In Azylis's case,
I know nothing. In fact, no one knows anything. Not the doctors, not
the specialists, no professionals of any kind. The bone marrow transplant changed the course of events. We intervened in the process. The
illness isn't progressing as it usually would. We've lost the map.

When, almost two years after the bone transplant, we noticed the
first symptoms in Azylis, we immediately turned to the team monitor-
ing her progress. We wanted to know what these signs meant for the
future. And that was when we received an answer that you rarely hear
from a doctor: "I don't know." Azylis is actually the first child in France
to receive a bone marrow transplant at such a young age for this sort of
pathology. The medical professionals don't have the experience to know
what the future has in store for her. They're opening new doors along

with us, and discovering the effects of intervention with us. They're sharing in our hopes and disappointments.

I wished we could have had confident, precise answers to our questions, but I respect the candor of those doctors who came straight out and admitted the limits of their knowledge. They're not hiding the truth from us. They tell us what they know and recognize what they don't. And that only increases our trust in them. But it's so hard not knowing, perhaps even harder than knowing the truth. With Thaïs, we knew. We knew that there was no hope of saving her or even of prolonging her life for however short a time. So we gathered all our strength and went with her on her journey for the few months she had left.

The situation with Azylis is different. We don't know whether the illness will follow its trajectory slowly and inexorably, or whether it will stabilize. Will Azylis also have a brief life, or will she live a long time? I'd like to know so that I can be better prepared. You don't do the same sort of training for a sprint and a marathon. Which is why, now more than ever, I concentrate on the day at hand. I take one day at a time alongside Azylis. I live through today so that I'm better prepared for tomorrow. Because only the future itself will show us what her life is to be. But her life is written just from one day to the next.

I watch Azylis playing in her bath, lying in her specially adapted sling. I notice how she tries to grab the little red boat and ply it into the water. I listen to her laugh when she succeeds, encouraged by her brother's cheers. And I wonder: what's left of our hopes now? There's nothing left now of the hopes of a cure fostered by the long months after her transplant. Barely the memory of them. Perhaps just a vague impression. On the other hand, the hope of seeing our daughter happy is still intact. Better than that: it's incontrovertible. I see evidence of this every day in the smile she greets us with in the morning, and the one she leaves us with when she goes to bed at night. How does Azylis manage to be so happy? Her daily life has been difficult since she first arrived. She's constantly waging battles, accepting defeat, winning a few victories. I think the secret to her luminous smile goes back to her very first days, to the moment when we decided to take a chance on that bone marrow transplant.

THE PROFESSOR FINISHED HIS SENTENCE, ONE OF THE LONGEST HE'D ever spoken to us. He was not usually a man of many words, but he'd taken his time explaining the procedure for a bone marrow transplant, the expected benefits and possible risks. He charted the whole subject so that we were in possession of the facts when we made our decision. Loïc and I wished that we could have had a crystal ball to read the future and illuminate our choice. But we didn't have one. So there was only one question that really mattered: given the information we had and in view of the situation we were facing, what would be the best decision to reach on the spot? Not later, or the next day, but right then? We hardly had time to think. We didn't need to, anyway. We replied spontaneously, readily: we wanted to try to cure our daughter. This might seem an obvious choice to anyone not personally affected by the question. It was less so when we were in the thick of it. The transplant could be fatal to Azylis, the doctor warned, because the process itself had aftereffects. On the other hand, it could all go well, prove extremely effective, and cure her. That was what we all hoped. It could also only partially modify the illness. We agreed to run these risks.

Just after that yes spoken in one—slightly shaky—voice, Loïc and I left the doctor who was already preoccupied with telephone calls, setting the wheels in motion for the transplant. We stood over the Moses basket and watched our baby sleeping. We could have been a fairy godmother and fairy godfather come to endow the newborn with gifts and wonders. I couldn't help but wish that I had a magic wand to give my daughter the vital missing enzyme. Instead, we leaned in close to her sleeping face. I felt her peaceful breathing on my cheek, and held my own breath before saying, "Azylis, we've just been told you're sick, and we've decided to attempt the impossible to make you better. What we want to tell you, more than anything else, is that we love you. We love you, whatever happens and whatever your life turns out to be. We love you for who you are, little princess."

That was nearly six years ago now. So much has happened since then, enough to fill several lifetimes. But ever since then, I lean down over Azylis every day without exception and tell her that I love her; I love her as she is. I say it a little forcefully when I'm tired of this difficult, complicated life. I say it with a quiver in my voice when I'm afraid of what the future has in store for her. I say it in a whisper when my voice is choked with emotion. I say it with a butterfly kiss, fluttering my eyelashes against her cheek, when I'm overwhelmed with love. However I say it, I make this declaration of love to her every day. And every day I watch her smile light up a little brighter. Because she's sure of our unconditional love. Surely that's the most beautiful way to love your child: to love unconditionally, just to love? The most beautiful way, but not the easiest. I had to experience Thaïs's fragility and Azylis's even greater vulnerability to understand that.

I remember how proud I was when, at just the age of three, Gaspard made out a syllable. I feel slightly ashamed to recall thinking, *My son can read at three. I've produced a genius. I'm so proud! I love him so much!* Well, Gaspard didn't learn to read at three, except for that one syllable, which was most likely a guess. He learned to read in first grade, like all the other kids. Just before the Halloween holiday of his first grade, he ran to see me one evening when I arrived home from work tired and preoccupied. He was hugging his little book to his chest like a treasure. He sat down beside me, opened the book at random, and stumbled his way through a sentence, following the words carefully with his index finger.

"You see, Mommy, I can read," he said, his eyes shining. "Are you proud of me?"

I didn't dare admit that deep down I was a little disappointed and had grown tired of waiting for this day in the last few years. Gaspard guessed how I was feeling from the detached way in which I replied. I'll never forget what he said.

"Do you love me anyway, Mommy?"

Why didn't I just praise his achievement? Why didn't I clap my hands when I heard my son read for the first time? Why didn't I just hug him without saying anything? I couldn't because I wanted more and better from him. I wanted him to fulfill all my expectations, surpass them even; I wanted him to realize the dreams I'd constructed when I was pregnant with him. My love was unwittingly conditional on his success. I now realize that, until then, I didn't love my children for who they were, with their strengths and weaknesses, their good and bad qualities. I loved them for who I wanted them to be. With a demanding, ungenerous love. Azylis couldn't read at three. She won't be reading at seven, either. She'll never read. I don't love her any less for that. Her aptitudes and abilities don't condition the love I feel for her. And therein lies the key to her happiness. She knows that, whatever happens, whatever she does or doesn't do, we will love her. That isn't a hypothesis; it's an absolute certainty. A certainty that means she can carry on with her life serenely and confidently, not worrying about failing or falling or reaching her limits. Of course, this apprenticeship in unconditional love has also benefited Gaspard and Arthur. I now love each of my children for who they are. Just for who they are. And for everything they are. I have a profound conviction that nothing could make them happier.

Iᴛ's ᴡᴀʀ, ᴊᴜsᴛ ʟɪᴋᴇ ᴇᴠᴇʀʏ ᴏᴛʜᴇʀ ᴅᴀʏ! Tʜᴇ́ʀᴇ̀sᴇ ɪs ʙᴀᴛᴛʟɪɴɢ ᴡɪᴛʜ a hairbrush while Azylis twists and turns her head in every direction. How can a little girl who takes such a coquettish interest in her appearance hate having her hair brushed that much? Yet, in a few minutes' time, she'll be parading around with her pretty braids. Should we see this as a psychological effect of the chemotherapy she had as a baby in preparation for her bone marrow transplant? She lost all her hair, which isn't much of disaster for a one-month-old baby. But who knows? No, I should recognize this as evidence of my daughter's robust character. Thérèse doesn't give up, using all sorts of tricks to achieve her aim. As a last resort, she uses the ultimate argument: "Quick, Azylis, we need to make you all pretty. Jérôme's on his way." And the wolf becomes a lamb, meekly succumbing to Thérèse's expert, rapidly braiding fingers. She's just securing the last hair-tie when the front doorbell rings. One short, sharp ring. The effect is instantaneous: Azylis breaks into her most dazzling smile. Her Prince Charming has arrived.

The moment Jérôme steps through the door, Azylis has eyes only for him. With a crease of her brow, she dismisses us all. Except him. She delights in this tryst four times a week, but Jérôme's visits aren't social calls. He's here to make Azylis work, to supple up her inactive leg muscles, relax her arms, and straighten her back. Whatever her beloved therapist puts her through, Azylis tolerates it with a smile. It's not just that she's receptive to his masculine charms; she trusts him.

Jérôme first came to our house five years ago. It was December 13; the sky had clothed itself in ashen gray, like our hearts. We'd come home from the hospital that day with Thaïs in our arms. A few hours earlier the doctors had told us that our daughter was now presenting the final stage of the illness. Nine months after we'd been told she had it. Nine tiny little months . . . in the same time it takes for a new life to grow in a mother's womb, Thaïs had declined. While we'd waited to hear the doctors' prognosis, Loïc and I had decided to bring our daughter home to live with us. And die with us. We wanted to be with her right to the end. We had the physical and moral strength to make that wish possible, but we didn't have the medical expertise. Thaïs's sickness meant that she needed nurses and doctors to calibrate her medications, monitor her vital signs, and evaluate her condition. She also needed daily respiratory therapy sessions.

The staff in the neurological unit at the hospital supported our decision. They had as much faith in us as we had in them. They agreed that taking Thaïs home was the right solution for our family. Which is why, in less time than it takes to say it, they had set up a Home Care team to back us up. It all happened very quickly. So quickly that I've ended up thinking that the team had anticipated our request so that the nurses' visits and the delivery of medical supplies could coincide with our return home. The organization was impeccable. All we had left to do was find a physical therapist, which is how we met Jérôme.

For a year and a week, a succession of nurses, doctors, and therapists came to our house. In the space of a few days they learned details of our private family life: our hours; our moods, routines, habits, and preoccupations; our untidiness; and the things we fussed about. Over the months we established our new normal and forged genuine connections. I admired the way they were with us. They managed to achieve just the right degree of intimacy, perfectly balanced between professionalism and humanity.

Keeping a cool head and a warm heart, that's all that matters in caregivers' attitudes toward a patient. A cool head to maximize their medical competence, and a warm heart to preserve their humanity, whatever the circumstances. That is how they keep their focus not on the condition but on the patient. Because it's always the person they're aiming to help.

I remember one day sitting in silence in the waiting room of a large hospital when a professor called repeatedly to see the "leukodystrophy with the transplant." I waited for him to call Azylis by name before standing up and saying that we were there. From the irritation on his face, I could tell that he thought that my attitude was just the quibbling of an oversensitive mother. I had no desire to annoy him; I just wanted to remind him that he had an appointment with a little girl—yes, she had leukodystrophy, and, yes, she'd had a transplant, but first and foremost she was a little girl. So, even if the appointment is medically motivated, it is still a human encounter and not merely an observation of a case.

Some caregivers bury their feelings beneath thick layers of cynicism, distance, and icy composure, perhaps so as to not suffer too much and, surely, to avoid becoming too attached to their terminal patients. The right degree of intimacy implies a certain perspective, which is not to be confused with cool detachment. Other professionals are not afraid to allow their feelings to come to the surface. Like the Home Care nurse who came on an emergency call out to see Thaïs when things were really bad. In reply to my desperate question, "How do you think she looks today?" she said, with obvious emotion, "Beautiful—I think she looks beautiful." That was all it took to soothe me, to help me forget the wildly fluctuating vital signs, and to appreciate, serenely, what really mattered: Thaïs as she was at that moment.

Loïc and I always made a point of acknowledging the humanity of caregivers. I remember the hospital nurses' tears the day we took Thaïs home for the last time. I also remember a comment from a friend who criticized their sensitivity with the killer words, "Why on Earth were they crying? It wasn't their child who was leaving. They should learn how to behave." But I liked their tears. I interpreted them not as misplaced sentimentality, but as proof of all the love they felt for their "Princess Courage," as they liked to call Thaïs, and all the sorrow they felt to think that they would never see her again. I comforted those nurses and cried along with them. I hugged each of them to me and thanked them for their professionalism in looking after Thaïs. And I thanked them for loving her.

When it came to Thaïs's funeral, we invited Jérôme and the nurses and doctors who'd cared for her to sit right behind us, in among the pews of family members. Because each of them had meant something in Thaïs's life. None of them cured her, but every one of them took care of her, with professional competence and affection.

The endless round of visits hasn't dwindled now. After a few months' respite, it started up again for Azylis. Of the many caregivers who looked after Thaïs, Jérôme is the only one to have stayed on. Most of them we've never seen again. Azylis doesn't need their care. She's called on professionals from a different, paramedical sphere: occupational therapists, psychotherapists, and so forth. But no Home Care nurses, no doctors of palliative care, no pain specialists. And I hope she'll never need them. The Home Care team may no longer be part of our day-to-day existence, but they are inscribed in the story of who we are. They have touched our lives. Left their mark on them. We will never forget them.

Azylis stopped talking several months ago now. Several months that, if you add them all up, are close to making a year. She lost the power of speech just after the ability to walk. At the time she could say a good hundred words, then every one of them vanished, leaving her lips forever. But you should hear her chattering away like a magpie the moment Jérôme starts tending to her! She talks avidly, and Jérôme commentates with interest on her outpourings. At first, their exchanges might sound absurd: Azylis's words are unintelligible. And yet Jérôme's answers aren't just on auto-pilot, any more than Azylis's babblings are meaningless. She knows exactly how to make herself understood. Like Thaïs, who knew how to say what she wanted when she was walled in silence. I remember that heavy sigh of hers, to which I'd instantly reply, "I love you, too, my Thaïs."

Azylis's language isn't quite the same as her older sister's was in her time. They each found their own way of communicating, without saying a word. Azylis modulates sounds, changes her facial expression, and accentuates her hand movements to tell us what she means. We've learned to decipher her language, not without difficulty, patience, and concentration. Of course, we don't have far-reaching debates with her, but we fully understand the basics of what she wants to convey. And if we're ever unsure of how to interpret her expressions, Gaspard and Arthur come to our aid. They're both "bilingual" and have completely mastered Azylis's language. In fact, Arthur insists that his sister can speak perfectly well . . . but just not in the same way as the rest of us.

From my bedroom I can hear Jérôme and Azylis's conversation in full swing, but it is interrupted by the entry-phone buzzer. I'm not expecting anyone. Could it be the occupational therapist? No, she's not coming 'til early afternoon. The caretaker? Unlikely—she slips the mail under the doormat, and, anyway, she doesn't need to use the entry phone.

"Hello, I have a delivery for you."

"I'll let you in."

The voice mentioned the name of a company in his preamble, but too quickly for me to catch it. I really must remember to have the entry phone mended; it crackles terribly.

Moments later, a man comes to the front door carrying a large parcel.

"Could you sign here and write down what time I delivered it, please?"

Intrigued, I take the piece of paper he hands me, and lean on the table in the hall to scribble what he's asked of me. I hand him back the receipt, and he checks it over.

"You didn't need to put the date, just the time."

"Sorry, I wrote it without thinking."

"Mind you, it's not February 29 every day. And not every year, either."

"Yes, that's true. Thank you. Have a nice day."

I step toward the door to close it, but the delivery man doesn't move. He seems in no hurry to leave. In fact, he looks keen to chat.

"Just think of it, a day that only happens every four years. Make a bit of space between two days and, bang, add in an extra one. I've never really got what it's for. Apparently it makes up for a mismatch in the number of seconds or something like that. I learned that at school, but that was a long time ago. A whole day hidden between two other days. It's like being on Harry Potter's platform 9¾, don't you think? You do know Harry Potter, don't you?"

I don't have time to reply before he carries on, so I just nod.

"Anyway, at the station . . . what's the place called now? Well, it doesn't matter, in this station, in between two of the platforms, there's another one, an invisible one: platform 9¾. The only people who can get onto it are wizards, and it takes them to the most incredible place. You never know, February 29 might also have its own secret world. A weird, slightly magical, totally separate world, and only people born on February 29 can go there. When they get to their birthday-that-doesn't-happen-every-year, all this wonderful stuff happens to them. It could be anything. On leap years, they spend the day just like everyone else. But the other three years, when everyone thinks their birthday's over before it's even started, squeezed out between February 28 and March 1, they sneak out in the middle of the night, and have this whole day that belongs to nobody but them. Everybody thinks people who are born on February 29 have a raw deal, but actually they're the lucky ones. I wish it had happened to me. My wife's expecting our first baby, but it's not due 'til July. Not a hope of her giving birth today. Shame. Okay, well, I'll let you get on."

"Bye. Have a nice day. And thank you for being so cheerful."

"You're welcome. It's better to laugh than to cry in this life. You have a good day."

I close the door.

"Who was it?" Thérèse asks, coming over.

"An angel disguised as a delivery man, I think."

It almost makes me forget to open my parcels, but I tackle the first one, the biggest. I follow the instructions to remove the cardboard packaging: it houses a magnificent bouquet of virgin-white roses. I bury my nose into their half-opened petals, and, closing my eyes, I inhale their delicate fragrance. I reach for the second parcel, which is wrapped in black and brown paper. I peel the wrapping off carefully, starting by removing the round sticker holding down the fold. Inside I find a big box of chocolates. My Achilles heel. I open the box straightaway. The veil of glazed paper scrunches in my hand; I marvel at the orderly rows and breathe in the appetizing smell. I can make out notes of grilled hazelnuts and roasted almonds. I pick out a smooth, domed chocolate and taste it. Pralines, my favorite. I guess who they're from even before reading the gift tag. Flowers in honor of her goddaughter Thaïs and chocolates to comfort me—I recognize this thoughtfulness and generosity as my sister Amicie's. She's not the first to make a show of support today: my parents called early this morning.

A little later, my older sister left me a tender message. I expect that Loïc has had calls from his family, too. Each of them means so much to us. And we know that we can count on them, in the good times and when the going gets tough.

I can't imagine more devoted parents than ours. They teamed up to give us the best possible support. When we were in Marseille for four months, they took turns to be with us. Then they made sure that they were ready to respond at the least sign of distress. They were always there, traveling right across France to help us. They didn't count the miles, or the exhaustion, or their age, or their own heartache. They were in no way beholden, but they did it out of love for her and for us. They coped with our bad moods, our fears, our silences, and our ungratefulness. Or mine at least, because for a long time I had trouble accepting the fact that they shed more tears than I did. I find it hard to admit that without feeling ashamed. I knew that I wasn't the only one suffering, but I was convinced that I was the only one whose pain—a mother's pain—was legitimate.

Since Thaïs's illness, our two families have come together as one. Our respective parents have grown closer. They already had a lot in common, but they've developed a new connection, united by a powerful link: an ordeal. An ordeal that was aggravated by their double dose of pain: they bore their grief and ours. They experienced the agony of watching their granddaughter die in conjunction with the pain of watching their children suffer. I think that people often forget the grandparents' grief. And great-grandparents', too. My beloved Great Granny admitted to me that, with unhappiness, each step up the generational ladder experiences extra suffering. So when Thaïs died, she cried three times: once for her great-granddaughter, once for her grandchildren, and once for her children. And I like to believe that with happy events, she takes three times as much delight.

It took me a while to understand that I didn't have the monopoly on pain in this ordeal. No more than I have a monopoly on happiness, for that matter. None of us has exclusive rights to laughter or tears. We should never let anyone dictate how we express ourselves. Because each of us displays our feelings in way that fits our own personality, our strengths and weaknesses, our personal story, and our sensitivities.

I DON'T KNOW HOW I COULD HAVE FORGOTTEN—TODAY OF ALL DAYS. And I've walked across the living room several times already today, without thinking. But now this lapse on my part is staring me in the face. The small, gray console is still in shadow in the corner of the room. I can make out the unremarkable book resting on the fretwork stand. The edges of the pages are slightly yellowed and the corners curled. It's an old edition. It lived through the whole of the last century. I don't know what it's worth, but I know its sentimental value. That value lies simply in the title, whose five black letters stand out on the otherwise pale front cover: *Thaïs*. This book, by Anatole France, is a romanticized account of the story of Saint Thaïs, an exceptionally beautiful courtesan in fourth-century Egypt who was converted to Christianity by a hermit monk called Paphnuce. Despite the beautiful writing, this book is not considered significant in the teeming annals of French literature, but it caught my attention. And Paphnuce's name may have fallen into obscurity, but the name Thaïs has survived more than sixteen hundred years to come and inscribe itself onto my heart.

This book is the only allusion to my darling daughter. In front of the bookstand we've put a small tea-light holder with an image of a bird with outstretched wings. Every day I light a tea-light candle, one of those small, round, white candles in an aluminum holder that you can buy by the hundred. I put it in the middle of the holder and let it burn all day. Every day. Except today. I forgot. There's still time to make up for this absentmindedness. I go to find the matches and the bag of candles. It's almost empty; my stocks are dwindling fast. I take out one of the last tea-lights, strike a match, light the tiny wick, and wait a few seconds for the wax to start beading. I pick up the glass holder gently. Its neck is slightly blackened by the smoke from previous days, so I rub it clean with my finger. I drop in the candle and watch as it lights up the corner of the room with its gentle glow. The letters on the book cover behind it dance in the flickering flame. Anatole France's Thaïs seems to come to life. My Thaïs is no longer here, but this ritual honors her memory and means that she still shines in our lives.

"Mommy, you lit Thaïs's candle without me."

Arthur got here too late, and he's disappointed. He likes blowing out the match and watching its incandescent glow subside.

"I'm so sorry, Arthur. We can do it together tomorrow, okay? Anyway, you know what, we need to light more candles for Thaïs today because it's her birthday."

"Her birthday? Do you have birthdays when you're dead? I've never seen Thaïs's birthday, and I've never seen Thaïs," he says with a little pout of regret, but then his face brightens as he adds, "I've never seen Thaïs, but I know her."

And he's right. He's known Thaïs ever since he was tiny. Thanks to us. And, especially, thanks to Gaspard.

It was three years ago, but I remember it as if it happened yesterday. A few more seconds and I would be there; I couldn't wait to get into the apartment. My load wasn't heavy at all, but it was precious. Loïc had dropped me outside and had gone to park the car before joining me with the rest of the luggage. I wasn't very strong yet, just about able to get up to the apartment. I stood by the door rummaging through my purse, cursing because I can never find what I'm looking for, but I eventually extricated my keys. I opened the door with a sigh, "Phew, I made it." It felt so good to be home.

As I walked inside, I almost bumped into Gaspard, who was right behind the door. He was standing straight as a little soldier, waiting for me with a big smile, and with his hands, face, and knees covered in dirt. I looked down and noticed that his soaking-wet stud boots were leaving dirt on the parquet floor. It was a Wednesday. Gaspard was just home from rugby training. He hadn't wasted any time changing, for fear of missing our new arrival. He was clasping his hands in nervous anticipation, hesitating for a moment before rushing out his words all in one breath: "Hi, Mommy. How are you? Please can I hold him in my arms?"

I was still holding the little Moses basket in which Arthur was sleeping. I'd come straight from the maternity unit with my gorgeous, clean, pink baby.

"Well, it's just, um, I'm not sure that's a good idea. You've never held a baby. He's so tiny and fragile. And you're all wet and muddy. Maybe not now."

I couldn't bring myself to tell him that I was frightened of letting him hold the baby. Gaspard wasn't yet seven. He was more used to flooring his opponents on the rugby pitch and crushing the ball under his weight as he scored tries than carrying a newborn baby.

"But I'd really like to hold him, please."

"Oh, okay, but you'll have to sit down."

"No, that won't work. I want to show him around the apartment. I'm his big brother. I want to welcome him home."

This argument got the better of my reluctance. I gave in to Gaspard: he could carry his little brother if he went and changed, and washed his face and feet. Gaspard ran off into the bathroom, his perky whistling smothering the sound of running water. He reappeared a few minutes later, clean as a new pin and impeccably dressed. He'd even gone so far as to run a brush over his ill-disciplined hair. He reached his arms toward Arthur, waggling his fingers.

"It's okay, Mommy; you can give him to me now."

Still, I hesitated. Every day I had to force myself to learn to trust, and that day was no different. So I entrusted Arthur to his brother, but I couldn't help rattling off a litany of advice: "Be careful with his head; put your hand along his back; don't run when you're carrying him; don't make any sudden moves; don't shout in his ears; don't let go." A mother's fears are so difficult to restrain! But they didn't bother Gaspard, who took Arthur very gently in his arms. He talked to him softly and started showing him around the apartment. I followed closely behind, holding back my urge to intervene.

Gaspard went into the room that Azylis and Arthur would be sharing. He described the antique cradle with its drapes hanging from a swan-neck, and the changing table laden with lotions and creams. He explained that the cot in the other corner of the room was Azylis's, and the same went for everything in the room that was pink. He walked out of the room and arrived outside the next bedroom. Its door was closed, but Gaspard didn't open it.

"This is my bedroom, Arthur. It's a big boy's room with big boy's toys. You're not allowed in here. Actually, look," he said, crouching down. At the foot of the door, almost along the floor, he had stuck a No Entry sign.

"You see," he said, pointing at the sign, "it's written there. You can't say you didn't know. If you want to come in, you'll have to ask me."

I stifled my laughter. Gaspard still had a lot to learn about babies and what they could do! He continued his introduction to the apartment in the same vein, glossing quickly over rooms he didn't deem of interest to his little brother: the toilet (he was in diapers), the kitchen (he was breastfed). They ended up in the living room and sat down on the sofa, Gaspard settling himself comfortably with his back firmly against the backrest and a cushion under his arm supporting Arthur. I went over to take my baby back.

"Wait, I haven't finished. I want to tell him something now. Could you leave us, Mommy? This is a brother thing."

I didn't know what to do with myself. I was intrigued by Gaspard's request, but I understood that this was between them and not for me. So I left the room and hovered in the doorway, in earshot. I was curious to know what the two of them had to share.

Gaspard cleared his throat, adjusted Arthur securely in the crook of his elbow, and began seriously, "Okay, so you know the apartment. And you know our family. You saw Mommy and Daddy right after you were born. Then Azylis and me came and visited you, with Thérèse. So that's your family, but there's also somebody you can't see. Actually, no one can see her anymore. It's Thaïs. She's dead. Do you know what dead means?" Silence. "Okay, it doesn't matter if you don't know. Thaïs is your sister, bigger than Azylis but not as big as me. I'm going to tell you about her life so you know her."

I leaned against the wall with all my weight to stop myself from sway-ing. I hadn't yet spoken Thaïs's name in front of Arthur. I hadn't dared. But now I listened and absorbed Gaspard's words. He talked calmly, describing Thaïs's arrival, how happy he was to have a little sister, but also his fear that she might steal our love away. He talked through her first two years, a time of perfect happiness. He admitted to all the tricks they'd gotten up to together, and those she'd undertaken on her own. I learned a few I hadn't known about. I smiled as I pictured my daughter climbing onto a stool on top of chair to reach the candy jar, or soaking her book in the blue-tinted water in the toilet, and scrub-bing off her scribbling with a nailbrush. Gaspard mentioned their games of hide-and-seek and the outlandish places Thaïs found to hide: in the laundry basket, under the Christmas tree, inside the kitchen garbage can . . . he laughed as he described all this, but then his voice darkened. He tackled the news of her illness, remembered the tears we shed. Then he described his sister's symptoms and her gradual decline. He quite openly explained her infirmities, her struggles, the faculties she'd lost. At the same time, he put across the complicity between them, their games and secrets, how they roared with laughter, and how they cuddled. He described the little girl she was right up until the last day of her life, right up until the last sigh: her joy, her trust, her smile, the way she loved, her pure heart, her child's soul. And he concluded with this unlikely and unforgettable line: "You see, Arthur, Thaïs had a wonderful life."

There was no other sound, just Gaspard's voice, clear in the sur-rounding silence. I don't think I breathed through the whole thing. I managed without air so that my breathing wouldn't get in the way of hearing. Now I held back my sobs and let my tears fall silently. Under my breath I repeated his words: "Thaïs had a wonderful life." I'd never dared say it, afraid that people would be shocked or think me mad. Gaspard had said it so simply, so candidly. And it was true. Thaïs had a wonderful life.

A wonderful life . . . but so far from the picture that the phrase conjures. Far from the usual paths that invite us to grow, make quick progress, and live to a ripe old age. They urge us to develop our tendencies, hone our abilities, add to our experiences. Thaïs's life went against the flow; she started regressing. Shortly after she turned two and that memorable birthday, her condition worsened, irretrievably. In the ensuing months she stopped walking and lost her hearing, the power of speech, her eyesight, and the ability to move at all. By Christmas she'd reached the terminal stage of her illness.

I remember the warning words of one caregiver: "At the end of her life, your daughter will be just a beating heart." I'd found the words creepy at the time. They encompassed all the regressions we would have to cope with, insinuated everything that would be lost. They belittled Thaïs, reducing her to the involuntary beatings of her heart. But now I can appropriate that comment in my own way, modifying it slightly and asserting proudly that at the end of her life Thaïs really was a beating heart. Just a beating heart, not in the sense of a vital organ throbbing in spite of itself, but a heart beating as a universal, living symbol of love. Yes, in the last few months of her life, all Thaïs did was love and be loved. As a little girl at the age of barely three, she lost a lot in order to gain even more, sustained by all the love she received and enriched by all the love she gave.

And it is that beating heart that Arthur knows, thanks to everything we've told him about his sister. And thanks to the feelings he has deep inside his own heart.

MEN PROBABLY DON'T REALIZE THIS, BUT MAKEUP AS AN ART IS all about subtlety. Brightening the complexion, exaggerating the eyes, bringing out the kissability of a mouth, concealing flaws, and doing all this without it being obvious. Every woman has her own habits and little tricks. I won't spend long in front of the mirror today; a few moments for a dash of eyeliner, a dusting of powder, a touch of lipstick, and a drop of powdery perfume. I have a date with a man who knows me and loves me without makeup. A man from whom I can't hide anything. A man with whom I share my pain and my joy. Loïc. The love of my life for the last thirteen years. And for many more to come.

I remember that beautiful night. One of the shortest of the year, and the deepest, too, the eve of the summer solstice. A magical night that started in festive spirit. Damien, a childhood friend of mine, had organized a big party, for no better reason than the pleasure of getting us all together before people went away for summer vacations. He chose as his rallying point the town we all had in common, Berry in central France. He invited the regulars, the inseparables, the inevitables, and others I didn't know. A June evening when we were all so young, happy, and carefree. And lucky, too, because misfortune had spared us, so far.

It was a wonderful party. I was twenty-five, tripping lightly through a carefree life, and dancing, dancing, dancing . . . 'til I was dizzy. Out of breath and red in the face, I stepped out of the buzzing house into the coolness of the garden. It was so peaceful outside, with a few people chatting around tables lit by colored Chinese lanterns. I sat down on my own a little way away to savor a quiet moment. Snatches of muffled conversation drifted over to me, punctuated by peals of laughter.

Three friends and a young man I didn't know came to join me. They told me about a recent trip to Italy; I was meant to have gone with them, but a series of unforeseeable obstacles had made that impossible. I felt a little put out by the conversation, and joined in with a hint of disappointment. The young stranger didn't seem to be listening to what we were saying, but then he turned to me and asked, "Would you like to go to Italy?"

"Yes, I've always dreamed of it."

"I'll take you there one day."

And that was the end of the exchange. I'd spoken only a few words, but my head was spinning, and my heart was thumping in my chest. I forgot the noise of the party and the clinking of glasses, the conversations around us and the balmy evening, the full moon and the twinkling stars. Nothing mattered now but those hitherto unfamiliar eyes with their incandescent intensity as they stared into mine in the dark. I couldn't tear my own eyes away. I instantly knew, in the time it would take a lightning bolt to streak across the sky and strike the ground, that I would follow this man to the ends of the Earth.

It was definitely what they call a lightning strike. It happened to me, yes, me, who didn't believe in it, or at least jeered at all that nonsense. I'd always thought that love at first sight was just a romanticized version of two people meeting, fit only for fairy tales and fuelling the dreams of sentimental young girls. I didn't believe in Prince Charming, either, someone too perfect to be real . . . yet, with just one look, Loïc had won my heart. And his own heart didn't put up much resistance, either. A love like that should last forever, because it was shared, because it was authentic, and because it was so self-evident. Because it had dictated itself to us.

Bolstered by this conviction and blissfully in love, we brought our lives together before the altar barely a year after that idyllic meeting.

Our "happy ending" was well on track; we would live happily ever after and have lots of children. Everything conspired to make it happen: our love for each other, Gaspard's birth, then Thaïs's two years later, and our relationship wasn't darkened by stormy arguments or showers of tears. Until that August afternoon, until that beach in Brittany, until that funny little footprint of Thaïs's. Until that grain of sand in the cogs of our happiness, until that tidal wave on the peaceful shores of our existence.

You don't need to look at the statistics to know that a child's illness sounds the death knell for a disproportionate number of relationships. There was no reason why ours should be any exception to that rule. Loïc and I were made to be happy together, not to suffer. Even so, when we were told that Thaïs had leukodystrophy, our first reaction was a belief that our marriage wouldn't falter as a result of it. We were sure of our love.

Is loving each other enough, though, to face the storm? Is believing in those feelings enough to not waver? I don't think so, or I no longer think so. We were so convinced that our relationship would be safe through the ordeal that we didn't really look after it properly. First and foremost we were parents, caregivers, and nurses, too, at the expense of being two people in love. Which is why, without any major crises or specific arguments, we started to grow apart. Good Breton sailor that he is, Loïc understood the risks of slowly drifting. Unlucky the over-confident captain who sleeps at the helm and gradually slips off course, one degree at a time, without even realizing it. Unlucky the lovers who, too sure of their feelings, stop looking in the same direction, without even realizing it.

One morning Loïc and I woke up side by side like two strangers. For many long months we'd forgotten to spend time together as a couple, to look after each other and listen to each other. To love each other.

It was a painful realization, and there was a strong temptation to give up; we didn't feel that we had the strength to tack close to the wind by setting off together again. But someone else's words, which we'd come across some time before, made us reconsider the situation: when a couple celebrating their sixty-fifth wedding anniversary were asked the secret of this longevity, the elderly lady with her white hair and creased face seemed almost surprised by the question and replied, "We were born at a time when, if something was broken, you didn't throw it away; you fixed it." Loïc and I still wanted to believe in that world. Our boat was taking on water; we wouldn't stand by and watch it sink. We would plug the hole and bail. We were going to do something to save our relationship.

What was left of our incredible lightning strike? There was still a spark, only a tiny spark, granted, but, in spite of everything, it was a promise of warmth and comfort and light. We were free to let it die or tend to it and allow it to glow brightly once more. We reached the decision that day to do whatever we could to keep our love alive. I felt a bit like the Cro-Magnon man who found fire and worked to keep it alight. We were now responsible for this flame sent from the heavens. The flame that brought us together.

Our relationship as a couple was what kept our family balance. Now it had become our primary concern. I remember one spring afternoon when Loïc and I had decided to allow ourselves a few hours' escape from the house, so that we could take a deep breath and recharge our batteries. The last few weeks had been testing and exhausting, and things weren't that good between us. So we wanted to make the most of the first warm rays of sunshine to go for a walk as a couple. Loïc had come home for lunch; we'd just finished eating and were getting ready to leave, leaving the girls with Thérèse, when the nurse came for her daily visit. She spent a few minutes with Thaïs and came into the living room and announced, "Thaïs isn't doing very well today. Her heartbeat and respiration are erratic."

"Do you think it's serious?" Loïc asked.

"I don't know, maybe not, but it's hardly reassuring. I can see you're about to go out. Wouldn't you rather stay here?"

"Look, I know this isn't very good timing, but we're not doing too well, either," I confided. "We need to get out of here and spend some time together. We're not going far or for very long; we just need to catch our breath together."

"I totally understand," she replied without a moment's hesitation. "You're right to look after yourselves. I'll stay here with Thaïs while you're out. Don't worry about a thing; I'll be here. And I'll call you if anything happens. You have a lovely walk and make the most of it!"

We left with our minds at ease. Thaïs was feeling better when we came home. And so were we.

There's one thing I'm sure of now: loving someone for the rest of your life depends on making that decision over and over again. With or without a lightning strike. It depends on a decision that involves being prepared to take action. Because love is nurtured by action. Loïc and I have been invited for interviews and presentations together several times; on one of these occasions someone asked how our relationship withstood our ordeal. Loïc replied in a flash, "Our relationship is still good . . . for now!" My, was I surprised—no, dumbfounded—by his reply! It could have heralded the beginnings of a confession, or the end of a marriage. But Loïc treated me to a reassuring smile and an amused twinkle in his eye as he went on: "When I woke up this morning, I resolved to love my wife. To love her today, just for today. Right through 'til this evening. And when the twelve strokes of midnight have struck, I'll renew my decision for the next day. And I'll carry on like that every day of my life."

Yes, love itself may be the heart's inclination, a beat of the heart over which we have no control, but loving is a choice, and every new day is part of its apprenticeship.

THE KITCHEN IS FILLED WITH THE SMELL OF THE BEST DAUPHINOISE potatoes in the world, as made by Thérèse. It's creamy, melt-in-the-mouth comfort food. I'm almost regretting my decision to eat out. Thérèse has given me her recipe several times, but I can never make it quite the same. I faithfully select the ingredients and respect the order in which to make the dish, and the time it takes to cook. To no avail.

Thérèse, Azylis, and Arthur are already sitting at the table. Quite the connoisseur, Arthur has asked for a double helping right away, and is piling huge spoonfuls into his mouth while keeping up a stream of enthusiastic comments. Next to his, Azylis's plate is a sorry sight: it's almost empty. She doesn't eat very much anymore; over the last few months we've watched her appetite dwindle, and found meals dragging on for ages. As soon as she started to lose weight, we took action. We didn't hesitate for a moment, not this time. We contacted her doctor and asked him to give her a gastrostomy. I don't think a neurology team had ever seen such determination to have one fitted; it's an intervention that families usually dread. We knew all about it, having been through it with Thaïs in far more difficult circumstances when we'd avoided the truth for too long.

Every mouthful had become dangerous for Thaïs; it could have gone the wrong way and ended up in her windpipe. Thaïs was in a critical condition, and we hadn't even noticed. We hadn't noticed because we didn't want to accept that she needed an artificial feeding system. We were in denial about our daughter's decline. But there was no hope of any natural improvement, so we grudgingly agreed to a gastrostomy, and never regretted the decision. Thaïs quickly gained weight and some of her spirit, and meals were an enjoyable family get-together once again.

Informed by this experience, we didn't waste any time with Azylis. We preempted the situation to avoid having to make hasty decisions in stressful circumstances. Azylis needs strength and calories to grow and develop. Feeding through a gastrostomy gives her everything she needs and doesn't cost her any effort. Nutrients are delivered directly to her stomach thanks to a "button," which can be connected to a pouch of specially formulated milk. It's practical, discreet, and painless. In the early days Arthur thought that we were attaching the tube to his sister's navel. He tried in vain to imitate this and was distraught that it wouldn't work, convinced that his navel wasn't functioning properly. Gaspard then explained to him how the gastrostomy worked, mentioning that Thaïs had had one. Arthur pretended to understand with an "Oh, I see, it's just for girls, then."

Azylis still sits at the table with us, because she still likes food. She can eat a bit, but only things she likes. Pasta shells, fries, cheese triangles, chocolate spread—her menus would give most nutritionists and educationalists a heart attack!

Thérèse is busy cutting up the slices of potato into tiny pieces and crushing them with her fork. Azylis swallows each mouthful slowly. I kiss her gently and then go over to Arthur, unable to resist the temptation of stealing some food from his plate. He frowns at me to show his disapproval as I give him his kiss.

"Bon appétit, my darling. See you later."

"Where are you going?"

"I'm going to have lunch with Daddy."

"And you're not wearing a shiny princess dress?"

"No, not today," I say, smiling as I imagine walking into the restaurant dressed like Cinderella. And why not, another time?

The elevator is waiting for me, and I step into it. I press the button for the first floor and then automatically reach my hand toward another button, but stop myself. I was about to press the button to close the door, the one with two arrows pointing toward each other. Why this urge for the elevator to move straightaway? Gaining a few short seconds won't make any difference. I'm not in a hurry; I'm not late. But the urge is incredibly strong.

I read recently that this button is actually the most frequently used in elevators, far more than the one that makes the doors stay open a little longer to let more people in. We can't bear waiting. The hours in a day have to be used effectively, so these transitional moments are perceived as having no value. They impose an intolerable inactivity on us. We try to cut them as short as possible or to fill them to make the most of them. A few years ago, I decided to imitate Thérèse and stop chasing every last minute, to release the constant pressure I was unconsciously putting myself under. Thérèse instinctively lives like that. She has retained something from her African homeland, her Senegalese roots: an ability to relativize time and never to count it. She's not bound to clock-watching. She lives each moment as it comes, and appreciates it for what it is: a moment in her life. I want to take the time to live, and to live in the present like her. But our reflexes are thick-skinned. If I'm asked, "What are you doing?" I've so often replied impatiently, "Nothing; I'm waiting." How can I think like that? Waiting isn't doing nothing. Is there actually ever a moment when we do nothing? Nothing at all? Even thinking? At times we can say that we're not undertaking anything tangible, concrete, or worthwhile. Well, I now like the privilege of those moments because they afford me the luxury of apparent inactivity.

I'M NOT GOING VERY FAR. LOÏC AND I HAVE ARRANGED TO MEET IN the next *arrondissement* of Paris, in a place full of shared memories. The Métro would be the quickest way to get there, but I opt to take the bus. The air is cold, sharp, and crisp, with sunbeams brightening the mood. You'd almost think it was going to snow. I feel like mooching around and seeing something of the city, so the bus is perfect.

I choose a seat facing forward, by the window, and sit down with my purse on my knee and my forehead pressed against the cool glass. An ancient radiator is gasping out heat as best it can under my seat. The elderly lady beside me complains about it, afraid that the hot air won't do the circulation in her legs any good; she decides to move.

From one stop to the next, the bus trundles through my neighborhood. I never weary of it, and I say a silent thank-you to whoever planned this itinerary, perhaps without even leaving his office, so that it doesn't take the shortest route. The main arteries don't have the same charm as adjacent side streets do. My eyes glaze over, hardly seeing the paved streets, sidewalks, and buildings. A young woman's face appears in my mind's eye. I don't know her name; in fact, I don't know anything about her. I came across her yesterday evening, at the end of a talk. After listening to my account of my experience, she stood up to speak, clearly moved as she clutched the microphone. She asked shrilly, "How did you do it? How did you cope with what you went through? Are you some kind of superwoman? Do you have a magic formula? I can't think of anything more terrifying than my child being ill and dying. I couldn't live like you do. Actually I don't think I'd be able to live at all." I so understand her questions and her fears! I felt exactly the same before, just before all this happened.

I remember a comment someone made to explain the catastrophe that had struck us: "This has happened to you because you have the strength to bear it." Is that really right? Are ordeals meted out to us in relation to our ability to cope with them? If that's the case, I'll come right out and say that I'd much rather have been unable to triumph over the least little difficulty. Yes, I'd prefer to have been stripped of any strength, and to have kept my princess with me for life. I've thought a lot about that comment, and I definitely don't believe that our own abilities expose us to suffering proportionate ordeals.

I have no particular aptitudes; I'm not cut out to be a superwoman. And Loïc doesn't have a superhero costume, either. There's nothing exceptional about either of us. On the other hand, like everyone else, we have unsuspected strength. In fact, I'm totally convinced that we all have abilities that we don't even know are there. Some form of courage, resistance, endurance that we don't know about, but is revealed when we are tested. In extraordinary circumstances we're all capable of extraordinary strength. We draw on what we need from within ourselves. And our inner resources are far richer than we think.

Take, for example, the victims of natural disasters: earthquakes, tsunamis, and volcanic eruptions strike at random and affect vast populations. It's not as if the most valiant people are gathered together in one place beforehand. And yet, just think how many individuals go on to surpass themselves to survive. They forget their fear, their pain, and their limitations to obey a single urge: a love of life, a very effective motivation, a survival instinct. Think of the mothers running breathlessly with their children in their arms, men lifting impossible weights to free their loved ones trapped underneath, children surviving for days and nights with no food or water, and families rebuilding their devastated homes and putting back together their broken lives without a murmur. There's probably nothing incredible about these people in their steady, day-to-day lives. But, confronted with the worst, man has it in him to do his best.

I myself have survived a tsunami; I'm still reeling from the initial shock of the disaster, dazed by all the effort I've expended, convalescing from the accumulated exhaustion. For many months I pushed myself beyond my limits in order to confront an unimaginable situation. Until then I'd enjoyed the comforts of a well-ordered schedule; I'd never coped well with lack of sleep and had never liked hospitals. I forgot all that. I no longer count sleepless nights, days spent in hospital departments, alterations to my routine, or the setbacks I've sustained. All that time I waged battle on two fronts with different aims at stake: adding life to Thaïs's days, and adding days to Azylis's life. And carrying on living. I let myself be buffeted by the constant undertow of the waves; I often took a whole lungful of water, and more than once I touched rock-bottom, but I always made it back to the surface.

When I'm asked now how I managed to deal with it all, I say, with total honesty, "I don't know." Like so many of us, I was frightened of illness; like so many of us, I was convinced that I couldn't survive the death of a child. My first reaction when I was told that Thaïs had leukodystrophy was astonishment . . . that I myself was still alive. I thought that my heart would give out, struck down by the news. I'd like to quote Nietzsche to explain the unthinkable: "That which does not kill us makes us stronger." Given that I didn't succumb to that first diagnosis, I decided to face up to it, and by throwing myself into battle, I released superhuman strengths I hadn't previously demonstrated. They didn't abandon me once calm was restored, but returned to their silent and unobtrusive state.

If anyone ever tells me that they "can't do it" or "couldn't have done it," I always say, "You don't know; you can't know what you're capable of." And I tell them that they should summon up one special strength, just one: the strength to believe.

L OÏC IS NEVER LATE. I CHECK MY WATCH AND WALK A LITTLE FASTER: I'd like to get there before him so that I can watch him arrive, see him from a distance without his realizing it, and feel my heart swell at the sight of him. I turn the corner of the street and screw up my eyes to make out the front of the restaurant. I can see that familiar silhouette, leaning against his scooter, helmet wedged under one arm and phone pressed up to his ear: he's already there. I recognize his leather jacket, patinated over the years, his perennial jeans, and the beginnings of stubble casting a bluish shadow over his cheeks.

It feels like a long time ago now when Loïc used to get dressed every morning in a dark suit, a sober tie, a spotless shirt, and polished shoes. The days when he worked in swanky offices for prestigious clients, the consultancy days. The change came about right here, in this very restaurant, nearly four years ago.

We'd made a date to have lunch together, just the two of us. An unforgettable lunch. Loïc arrived first, and I noted with pride how elegant he looked in his well-cut suit, but as I drew closer, I knew immediately that something was bothering him. I could see it in that darkening of his eyes and the clenching of his jaw. He didn't speak until we'd been seated at our table. He ordered an aperitif, drank it down in one gulp, and blurted, "I want to talk to you about something." I didn't like the nervous note in his voice and was afraid he had bad news. Loïc took a deep breath before continuing.

"I want to change jobs."

Phew, if that's all it was, there was nothing to worry about. His career had been clearly mapped out since he left business school. Did he now want to embrace new ambitions, move into a bigger consultancy firm, or take on a position with more responsibility?

"Great idea!" I said, smiling, feeling reassured. "What are you think-ing of doing?"

"Carpentry. I want to be a carpenter."

I put my glass back down awkwardly, eyes wide, the breath knocked out of me.

"Carpentry? You want to be a carpenter? That's a joke, right? Tell me what you're really thinking of doing."

"Carpentry."

There was no trace of nerves in his voice now. Loïc was calm again, and I was the one wriggling in my chair.

"Ever since school, my exams, my studies, I've followed a pre-established path, and—perfectly logically—it's got me to the position of consultant. I've been really happy for years, but now I want a change."

I could hear what he was saying and could feel the sincerity of his words, but I couldn't bring myself to accept it. This change of professional direction made my head spin. I didn't need it. That whole month of September I'd felt more than ever that I was driving blindly along a narrow mountain road. Thaïs was very ill; the end was drawing ever nearer. Azylis was starting to show worrying signs of the illness. It was already several months since I'd put my own work to one side to have more time to take care of them. I was struggling to stay connected to the outside world and keep pace with it. I didn't know where this adventure would take our family: I'd always seen Loïc's work as an indispensable source of security, and I don't just mean financial. It was the safety net that stopped me from crashing down; it set a rhythm to our days and weeks. It calmed me because it was at least one area where I had nothing to fear, no doubts. Every other aspect of our lives felt uncertain. So why change? Why start from the beginning again? And why do it now, in the eye of the storm? I didn't hold back my tears as I told him no.

"I'm so sorry; I don't want you to leave your job and become a carpenter. It would be crazy, and I can't take any craziness in our lives. I need order and peace. The job you have now is reassuring because it protects us from financial uncertainty and because I know you're good at it. And, anyway, you don't know anything about carpentry."

"I'll learn. I'll do whatever training's needed. I've already done some research. I can get onto a course really soon."

"But what for? You like your consultancy work, don't you? It seems fulfilling for you, it pays the bills, it gives you a social standing. Why be a carpenter? You might lose all of that, you know? Can't you settle for what you have?"

"No. I want to be free," he said simply.

"Free from what? From your schedules, your vacations?"

"Free. Just free."

Loïc wanted to choose his own path in life, following his own inspiration, far from economic constraints and social considerations. But I countered this wish for freedom with my fear—my fears. Fear of change, fear of the unknown, but also a fear that I would no longer be so proud of this elegant man.

I changed tactics and tried to play for time.

"Fine, but there's no rush. You don't have to make up your mind right away. Wait 'til our family circumstances have settled down a bit. Wait 'til things have calmed down. Then we can talk about this."

"Don't worry, my darling," he reassured. "I can wait if you want, for as long as it takes. You're right, there's no rush. We'll make the decision together. But one thing's for sure: today's no better or worse than another day to change. If we always waited for the perfect combination of circumstances, we'd end up never doing anything. True, our lives are particularly complicated at the moment, but we shouldn't let that paralyze us. We have to carry on living and making plans, and putting them into action."

I understood what he meant by this and the reasoning he was introducing. We'd been told more than nine months earlier that Thaïs could die at any moment. A matter of days or weeks. When she'd come home from the hospital the previous December, no one could have imagined that she would still be with us for Christmas, even less so at Easter. We'd lived through many emergencies and had believed that the time had come several times, but she'd held out. No one was venturing prognostics about her life expectancy now. With his usual candor, Gaspard quite often said, "You told me Thaïs would die soon, but she's still here. Are you really sure she's going to die one day?" Yes, her imminent death was a certainty, but we didn't know when it would be. Not the time, nor the day.

In the early days we'd prepared ourselves for the shock, and had gathered our strength to make a united front, watching over her day and night. To the point of exhaustion. Only then did we drop our weapons and lower our guard. We accepted that we couldn't know; we couldn't control this situation. There was a strong temptation to stagnate in that state of waiting, to have no plans of any sort. To suspend our lives. We had to grasp the fact that this time, those weeks and months weren't a respite for Thaïs; they were her life. And Thaïs wouldn't want us to put our lives to one side while she lived hers. It was a weighty responsibility for her, being the cause of her family's inertia. An inappropriate responsibility.

The best way to pay homage to Thaïs's life, then, was to get on with living our own. We found the courage to go for a vacation, to go out in the evenings, to visit friends, to do things and go places. Which meant that we wouldn't be starting to live again after Thaïs died; we'd simply be carrying on living.

Loïc's change of profession belonged to that thought process: carrying on living. It is echoed in this quote from Oscar Wilde: "To live is the rarest thing in the world. Most people exist, that is all." What I'd always loved about Loïc wasn't his smart suits and clean-shaven cheeks but his freedom. He emancipates himself from social pressures and pointless conventions. Loïc is a free man, and that freedom is a treasure.

It wasn't until we'd finished lunch and I'd made my way home through the driving rain that my thoughts had fallen into place.

I stopped under a porch to call him: "Go ahead! I'm right behind you. I'll go with you on this journey. I trust you, so go on—live!"

Four years later I'm now looking at an accomplished carpenter and a fulfilled man, a little worried about his responsibilities in his small company, but happy. I'm more proud of him than I ever have been. Because he didn't choose the easy route; he chose freedom.

Loïc is just finishing his phone call as I come over. He's frowning and looks preoccupied. I know that expression: he's not worried, just concentrating on something, totally focused on it. He's talking about the doors of a wardrobe, the runners for drawers. I hesitate before disturbing him during his conversation, but can't resist it. He hangs up as I put my arms around his neck and stop him speaking with a kiss. I stroke his stubbly cheek, surprised to feel how rough it is. Loïc hasn't had time to miss me yet this morning, but I'm very happy to be with him again.

We walk into the restaurant hand in hand. I like this place; it still has an authentic atmosphere of the big brasseries of old with a 1920s charm. We walk along the cavernous corridor from the street into the restaurant, and I cast an eye over the menu set in a tall copper stand. Baked eggs with fresh oyster mushrooms, house special fish soup, steak tartare on request, pot-roast beef—utterly traditional French cuisine with no frills or pretention. Now I'm feeling hungry! We tell the waiter who greets us that we've booked a table for two, and he asks us to follow him.

The large dining room seats a lot of people, and every table is occupied. The atmosphere is warm, noisy, animated; it might be unbearable if it weren't for the glass roof, a magnificent opening to the sky. I look up and contemplate that great expanse of glass letting in natural light. The restaurant rises up over three floors, and there are plants growing all along the wrought-iron balconies. Our table is at the far end of the second floor, in a quieter spot. Loïc moves more quickly than the waiter to pull out my red velvet chair for me. Then he sits down opposite me and gestures to the waiter not to go away. We order right away: medium steak, fries, and a glass of good red wine. We'll see about dessert later, but I have an idea in the back of my mind: I have fond memories of their rum baba.

Once we're settled, but without discussing it, we both put down our phones next to our folded napkins, then look at each other as we switch them to silent and stow them away, his in his pocket and mine in my purse. We don't want to be disturbed. This hour belongs to us, and us alone. Loïc and I have gotten into the habit of meeting like this regularly, as a couple. Time enough to go for a walk, have a meal, watch a movie; more important, time enough to escape the whirlwind of family life and work pressures. We just want to be together, that's all.

The conversation starts out gently, affectionately. We talk about everything and nothing, day-to-day things. About us, a bit. At the next table a couple are eating in silence. All you can hear is the metallic clink of cutlery, the chime of a glass knocking into the edge of a white porcelain plate. They look down and chew indolently. There's no feeling of animosity, only a worn-out quality that demonstrates the weight of years spent together, of habit and routine. Perhaps we would be like this, too, if circumstances hadn't woken us up, rattled us. The woman looks up and gazes at the room over her husband's shoulders, first the right and then the left, without stopping to look at his face, as if he were transparent. She catches my eye, and I smile at her. She glances furtively at Loïc's hand holding mine. From the sigh she gives and the expression in her eye, I can sense not sadness but disillusionment. She leans toward her husband and says something quietly; he barely answers. I squeeze Loïc's hand a little tighter. Let's love each other forever!

The waiter arrives with our order, sets down our plates, and fills our glasses with wine. He gives us a carafe of water and a basket of bread, then puts down the little steel holder with salt, pepper, and a small pot of mustard.

"Bon appétit," he calls as he walks away.

Our plates are laden with food, and we dig in straight away. I pick up a fry in my fingers; it's nice and hot and crispy. Before biting into it, I ask Loïc, "Do you remember Thaïs's birthdays? The ones we spent with her?"

"Of course! There were three of them . . . only three."

I can sense the woman at the next table straining her ears, so I carry on more quietly.

"Three birthdays, and they were all very different if you think about it."

Now that I put my mind to it, I realize that these landmarks for Thaïs really had had very little in common. We had a happy celebration for her first birthday, like so many other loving, carefree parents. I'd made a big cake to match her love of food. I remember how surprised Loïc was when I ran out at the last minute to buy more candles.

"But we have a whole packet. Why do you want more?"

"Because I want a pink one! I can't give my daughter a blue candle!"

From the indignation in my voice, Loïc knew not to persist. He gave in and, with half a smile, sighed, "Oh, you girls . . ."

We helped Thaïs blow out that pretty pink candle, thinking eagerly, "This will be the first of many birthdays."

The following year I'd prepared everything the day before: the cake, the presents, the decorations, and the white candles with pink spots, the ones that relight by themselves. But when D-day came, nothing went the way I'd planned. How could I ever forget her second birthday?

I STUMBLED ALONG THE CORRIDOR. LOÏC WALKED BESIDE ME, holding my elbow, his own stride far from steady. We made it out to the street like that, leaning against each other to stop ourselves from falling. We pushed the door open and stepped outside, hit by the late winter chill. I hadn't thought to button up my coat on the way out, and started shivering. Loïc pulled the woolen fabric around me and did up the buttons, then turned my collar up and drew me to him. The warmth of our bodies formed a single, unified rampart against the wind. Clinging to each other, we gradually, painfully, came back down to Earth. Minutes earlier our lives had been turned upside down. In the worst possible way.

It was March 1, and we had just learned that our little Thaïs had an incurable illness. We'd heard two words with the bleakest of implications, metachromatic leukodystrophy, for the first time. We'd grasped that Thaïs would soon die. I'd almost screamed at the doctor, "That's not possible; you've got it wrong. It's her birthday today! She's two years old." Two short little years, which actually already represented more than half her life.

Loïc and I hadn't exchanged a word since we heard the news. We stood there in the middle of the sidewalk, distraught. Nothing going on around us registered with us. We didn't feel as if we were there. It was as if our bodies had been dismantled, our cells had scattered, our minds had disintegrated. We were no longer us.

I opened my mouth to speak, and didn't recognize my own voice.

"Loïc, promise me we won't tell the children. Not right away, at least. Let's leave it as long as possible."

Loïc relaxed his grip and stood back to look me in the eye.

"You want to hide this from them? Why?"

"Because, more than anything else, I want to protect their innocence."

Is there anything more precious than a child's innocence? Gaspard was four and Thaïs only just two. What did they know about life's hardships? Nothing. That sort of thing had nothing to do with them. They were too young. I wanted to spare them so that they could live in a world of Winnie the Pooh and Babar the Elephant for as long as possible, in a place where there was no pain, no fear, and no death. They would come up against the harsh adult world soon enough. One day they would find out that not everything was pink and round and good. But not today. I was frightened that the news would damage them irreparably.

Loïc listened attentively to my plea, and his words were a gentle whisper in my ear when he replied, "What are we going to tell them, then? That everything's fine? And then go on as if nothing's happened? Hiding our pain and our tears? Pretending to laugh and smile? It's a high price to pay, and we may protect their innocence, but we'd lose their trust. Because they'll find out sooner or later. And rather sooner than later. They'll know the truth soon enough when Thaïs gets worse. And then they'll know we lied to them, and they'll never believe us again. I think nothing's more important than children's trust. Gaspard and Thaïs believe in us, more than anything else. What would we be protecting them from if we keep this quiet? From life? From their own lives? Because this is what their lives are, whether we like it or not. And, first and foremost, this is Thaïs's life. We have to reinforce the trust they have in us, and we in turn have to trust them. We're going to talk to them straightaway. I'm sure we'll cry, a lot, but we'll be crying together. We're going to get through this ordeal, and we'll get through it as a family."

I agreed, nodding my head again and again, but I didn't say a word, my throat knotted with stifled sobs.

We told Gaspard and Thaïs the truth that same day, with no pretense. We didn't mention metachromatic leukodystrophy or degenerative, genetic, neurological disorders, not wanting to hide behind these complicated terms to drown out the bare facts. We used words they could grasp so that they really understood. We explained that Thaïs had an illness, which meant that she couldn't do some things today and wouldn't be able to do others tomorrow. We told them that, because of this illness, she wouldn't live for very long, but we reassured her that, whatever happened, we'd always be there. We didn't silence our own tears while we told them, and Gaspard shed tears of his own. We stayed there together for a long time, united in sorrow.

With no warning, Gaspard eventually dried his tears with the back of his sleeve and asked, "Okay, so are we going to have Thaïs's birthday party now?"

"No, sweetheart," I replied, confused. "We're not going to have her party now. Do you understand what we just told you? We've been told your sister's sick. We're too sad to have a party."

But Gaspard wasn't going to be thrown that easily, and he turned to me with his clear eyes and candid smile to reply, "Yes, I totally understand. And I know she's going to die. But she's not dead now. And it's her birthday today. So why aren't we having a party for her?"

It was only when he took his sister by the hand and led her out of the room singing "Happy Birthday to you!" at the top of his lungs that I understood. I understood what childhood innocence was. It's not the not knowing. It's not growing up in blinkers so that you see only beautiful things, and then one day opening your eyes to all the pain and difficulty in the world. Children know, whatever we say about them and whatever we say to them. They don't understand events in their entirety as adults do, and they don't try to control them: they experience them as they come. And they have no trouble finding their way back to happiness—and taking us along with them. A child's innocence consists of knowing the truth and living with it quite naturally, without fear, without projections, just carrying on trustingly.

The day of Thaïs's second birthday, I realized that if I wanted to continue loving life and having my share of happiness, I had to rediscover the child in me.

I allowed that child in me free expression for Thaïs's third birthday the following year. We knew it would be our last birthday with her, but rather than wallowing in sadness, we decided to celebrate it twice, on February 28 and March 1, to make the most of it. We gathered around her in her bedroom; Gaspard climbed onto the bed to be right next to her, and Azylis reached out her arms toward her sister. We sang a loud, hearty "Happy Birthday," exuberantly celebrating the year we'd just had rather than thinking about the year that lay ahead and the pain it heralded. We cooked cakes she didn't eat, chose presents she couldn't open, and invited friends she couldn't see. Thaïs was at the party in her own way, her own subtle and discreet way. With the hint of a smile, the depth of a sigh, the glint of an eye, she let us know she was happy. And we were, too. We were so happy along with her.

I'M STRUGGLING TO FINISH MY PLATE, AND I SIT THERE THINKING about the past a while longer. Loïc brings me back by stroking my cheek, wiping a discreet tear from my eyelash. Then he picks up his glass and raises it toward me in a toast.

"To us. To her. Happy Birthday, pretty princess!"

"Happy Birthday."

The neighboring couple are paying their check, and Loïc attracts the waiter's attention with a wave. He orders two coffees, then hesitates.

"Or did you want a dessert?" he asks me.

"No, thanks, I've eaten plenty. That was perfect."

"What about that rum baba you were so tempted by?"

"Another time."

"So, two coffees, then. One espresso and one Americano."

Loïc knows me well; he knows that really strong coffee upsets my stomach. It's an aftereffect of the difficult years: neither the body nor the mind emerges unscathed from life's painful experiences. For more than five years now I've had trouble with heartburn and muscular tension in my back, just below my left shoulder blade. As for the bruises on my heart . . .

The woman next to us stands up to follow her husband out. As she passes me, she says, "I heard it was your birthday, so Happy Birthday!"

"Actually, it's not my birthday, but thank you anyway."

"I'm sorry," she says, embarrassed. "I thought you were celebrating a birthday."

"Yes, it's our daughter's birthday."

"Oh, okay. How old is she?"

"She would have been eight."

She stands there speechless, her mouth hanging open and her cheeks flushed.

"I'm sorry. Really so sorry. I . . . I should have minded my own business. But I couldn't have known. It doesn't show . . . you look happy!" she exclaims, and leaves before we have a chance to say anything.

How many times have we heard that comment? People seem amazed that what we've suffered hasn't left some indelible trace on our faces. Does emotional pain leave scars? Does suffering produce wrinkles? Do tears leave tracks? Sorrow reddens my eyes, drains my cheeks of color, and pinches up my mouth, sometimes several times a day. But it doesn't last; when it leaves me, it takes the mask of sorrow with it, giving way to the sparkle of life once more.

The ordeals we've been through don't summarize our whole life. They are a part of it, of course, and they have a significant role in our day-to-day concerns, but they haven't contaminated every aspect of our existence. This reminds me of a man I came across on the beach when I was a little girl. He was a friend of my parents, and he spent his summer vacation in the same place as us every year. He had an arm missing; it had been amputated after a serious injury during the war. The first time I met him, I remember that I couldn't take my eyes off that scarred stump and the absence beneath it. I focused on this missing limb. The man had other physical characteristics—he was tall and athletic—but that was the only thing I noticed about him. For me he was "the man with the missing arm."

I constantly asked my father about him. He must have been in terrible pain at the time of the accident, and worse psychological pain when he was told that the arm would have to be amputated. He must have struggled to get through the early days. So much to cope with: tending to the wound, rehabilitation, other people's reactions. Eventually he'd accepted this new life and adapted to his situation. He'd returned to work, resumed his sporting activities, and even drove the same car. He didn't pretend to ignore this distinguishing feature, any more than he drew attention to it. After spending a few days with him, we all forgot his disability and saw him for who he was: a man, a husband, and a father. How many arms he had didn't alter that.

Two new people come to sit at the next table, and their serious expressions imply that they're here for a business lunch. Loïc and I finish our coffees, pay the check, and leave. Our seats won't stay empty for long; the restaurant is still just as full. Back out on the street, I ask Loïc whether he'd like to stay with me a little longer and go for a walk. He looks at his watch and hesitates for a moment before being sensible: it's too tight; he really needs to get back to work; he has a client waiting. So, sadly, I have to say good-bye. Before he puts his helmet on, I kiss him gently and say, "Ride carefully, and don't be home too late."

As Loïc rides off, I switch my cell phone back on, and the screen immediately informs me that I have several texts and a few voicemails. I run through them quickly: they all refer to Thaïs's birthday. I save them to savor them fully later, but I do listen to all of them, always afraid that there will be a call from Thérèse with bad news or asking me to come home as quickly as possible. It's already happened several times, especially since Azylis has started having epileptic fits. So I'm never completely at ease when I'm away from home, even less so when I can't be contacted. You never know what might happen.

Thérèse hasn't called, and I resist the temptation to call her. I adhere to the tried-and-tested formula of "no news is good news" and put my phone in the inside pocket of my purse. I look at the time, and I'm pleased to see that it's not that late, and I have a feeling that I very rarely have in my life, something I like more than anything else: I have some time to spare. Time just for me. Time I'd like to spend with her.

I KNOW ALL THE LITTLE SHOPS ALONG THIS STREET, PARTICULARLY THE shoe shops and fashion stores. They couldn't change a single sign without my noticing. With a bit of concentration I would even be able to list them in the correct order. I have to say that this is one of my favorite places, and I regularly plow up and down its sidewalks.

Today I have no trouble resisting the window displays as I walk purposefully down to the end of street. I rarely venture this far, usually concentrating my expedition at the top end near the over-ground Métro line. The purpose of my trip today is here at the bottom of the street, where the stores relinquish their hold. I keep walking, my eyes pinned on the building that stands tall and perfectly white on the far side of the crossroads. I glance right and then left, and almost run across the street. A driver sounds his horn to chide me for taking the risk. I should have used the nearby pedestrian crossing, but didn't want to divert my route. I apologize with a wave.

I've never been through these white gates flanked by two chestnut trees, currently in their winter nakedness. I reach the paved area in front of the steps and gaze up at the tall, pale stone steeple. Its finely wrought architecture is at odds with the simplicity of the rest of the building.

As if nineteenth-century builders gave preferential treatment to vertical structures and to that pinnacle touching the sky.

I climb the steps one at a time, in no hurry, counting them mechanically, and walk under one of the arches towering over the entrance. Then I turn around to enjoy the view of the busy street. It's a striking contrast: here, material things give way to the spiritual; noise eclipses itself in favor of silence. I open one side of the double doors and finally step into the building I've been drawn toward.

There is no service at this time of day; the church is peaceful and quiet. It is much larger than its façade implies. The nave with its vaulted ceiling supported by plain columns leads all the way to the choir. There are neat rows of chairs on either side. I walk over to them and stroke the satin sheen of their wooden backrests.

I can't count how many seats there are. The atmosphere must be very different when the nave and transepts are full of people. For now, half a dozen faithful souls are here in quiet prayer, absorbed in their personal meditations. Two women are standing beside a column in a side aisle, whispering to each other quickly. I choose a chair in one of the last rows and sit down gently to avoid making the rush seat creak. The lights are dimmed; only timid rays of February sun filter through the tall stained-glass windows. I look at the multicolored flecks that they project on the bare walls and the rough-hewn stone of the floor. Then my gaze is automatically drawn to the far end of the nave. A mural fresco lends its color to the curved wall behind the choir, without detracting from the restrained simplicity of the place. I close my eyes. It feels good to be here.

Churches were a refuge for me in my darkest hours. Wherever I was—in Paris or Marseille, in Brittany, Berry, or somewhere else—I often stepped through their doors in search of some inner peace and calm. I would sit quietly, far from prying eyes, as I am today. Plenty of times I went in crying and came back out comforted. I didn't come to be consoled but to abandon myself. To entrust myself. And to recharge the faith that fuels and illuminates me.

I've believed in God since I was a very little girl, and I believed with a peaceful, comfortable faith, which had so far not met with the trials of this world. I found it easy to believe when life smiled on me, to worship

God's goodness when it bestowed so many good things on me. It was all straightforward until Thaïs's illness disrupted my whole world, like a dog rampaging through neatly standing skittles. My horizon darkened that day. In a few moments, the future turned frighteningly bleak, cloaked in deep misfortune. I stopped myself from projecting into that future, stopped looking ahead, for fear of losing myself. I looked up toward the heavens, and tried to find the light.

Through all that ordeal, through my dizzying climb up my own personal Himalayas, my faith in God became my lantern or, to be more precise, my headlamp, the sort that mountain climbers wear in the center of their foreheads to help them see where they should put their feet to climb safely. This lamp lit the way for me, driving away the frightening darkness, so that I could carry on with confidence. Its beams didn't reach as far as the summit; they shed their light over the path I needed to follow, one foot after the other, through my daily life. No further than that. They made me concentrate on the day ahead, and not worry about my life as a whole. Yesterday has been; tomorrow will be; only today actually is.

Despite my conviction in my faith, I didn't succumb to my ordeal with docile apathy. How many times I screamed my fear and distress at the sky, how many times I wailed my weariness and anger! But not once—no, not once—did I rebel against God, nor against anyone, for that matter. Because I never asked myself, *Why?* I never asked for a reason behind any ramifications of my situation: *Why me? Why my daughters?*

I refused to go down the route of explanations and justifications. I sensed instinctively that I would get lost in the whys and wherefores. As a result, I've never felt that I was a victim of injustice, any more than I felt guilty of some misdeed. I didn't try to find something responsible for my misfortune. I could have easily accused God of meting out suffering from up on His cloud. What would have been the point? I don't need enemies to overcome my pain. I want allies, support. And God has proved to be an unfailing mainstay.

A few months ago I came across a text that has a parable-like quality. The title brought a smile to my lips: *Footprints in the Sand*. I see it as a gentle nod to Thaïs and her unforgettable little footprints in wet sand. There is no authenticated provenance for this text, although it is often attributed to the Brazilian poet Ademar de Barros. An inspired poet. It is about a man who dreams that he is walking along a beach with God by his side, and he sees all the scenes from his life scrolling across the sky. He views them one after the other and turns around to see that there are two clear sets of footprints in the sand behind him: his and God's, side by side. When he looks more closely, he notices that in some places there is only one set of footprints. These single sets correspond to the most difficult, worrying, and trying periods in his life. Deeply disappointed, he turns to God and asks Him why He abandoned him in the worst times, just when he needed support. The Lord replies that the exact opposite is true and that He never left him on his own, far from it. In times of difficulty and suffering, He was very much there; it is His footsteps that are left in the sand, leaving deeper footprints, because, when times were difficult, He was carrying the man on his back.

So, rather than trying to find a reason and a meaning, rather than going around in circles in search of a justification, rather than sitting on the edge of the path waiting for God to climb it instead of me and in my name, I decided to set off on my journey. Because it was my life. And it was up to me to live it. On the way I up, I continued to trust in God, as a child has faith in his or her parents. I knew that I would never face my trials alone.

A grieving mother once said to me, "I really envy you. It's easier for you to bear because you believe in God." I completely understand what she means, and yet . . . if she only knew how I've suffered! Her pain has nothing to envy mine. When the time came to say a final farewell to Thaïs, I felt the unfathomable agony of any mother losing the flesh of her flesh, believer or not. When the cold earth covered Thaïs's beloved body, I was in utter darkness; I lived in the shadows, like every mother who won't see her child again. Faith doesn't stop us from suffering. It isn't a panacea, a miracle cure against physical and emotional pain. It spares us none of our human sorrow, but it warns us against the terrible stumbling block of despair. I remember something Gaspard said a few weeks earlier, the frank, illuminating words of a child.

THE RACE WAS ON, AND I WAS STRUGGLING TO CATCH MY BREATH. Every time I picked up Gaspard from school he made the same request: "Can we race?" I mostly avoided the challenge, pointing at my feet, "I'm so sorry, darling, I'm wearing high-heeled shoes." But that day he wanted to measure up to me, and he'd anticipated my standard reply.

"I know you're wearing heels," he reasoned, "but I'm carrying a very heavy satchel. We're even. So, shall we do it? Come on, Mom; it's easy; it's downhill."

So I'd agreed this time, but I was regretting it now. I'd long ago adopted Winston Churchill's "no sport" edict, and it suited me very well. I'd have to remember not to forsake it again.

Gaspard was at the bottom of the hill several seconds ahead of me, laughing triumphantly as he waited. I joined him, panting, and put an arm around his shoulders.

"You're too quick for me. I can see why your rugby coach calls you the 'dynamo'!"

I'd accepted his challenge that time because I wanted to make him happy; I wanted him to be in a good mood.

"Gaspard, I have something sad to tell you."

"What? What is it? Mommy, tell me what's going on."

"Tiji's dead."

Tiji was my parents' dog, a beautiful Bernese Mountain dog. Gaspard had taken to him the moment he arrived and had even given him his name. My mother had called me that morning to tell me the news, and I'd immediately envisaged how upset Gaspard would be when I told him. I'd decided to tell him the truth straight out, the way he'd taught me a few years earlier, when he told me that I should use the word "dead" instead of hiding behind "He's left us," "He's gone," "He's no longer here," or "He won't come back." Children don't like euphemisms; they're not afraid of words. At the time Gaspard had spoken the unforgettable words: "Death's not a big deal. It's sad, but it's not a big deal." Informed by this experience, I'd now succeeded in telling him Tiji had died with no preamble. It was small victory, but I was proud of it.

Gaspard didn't say a word. His face drained of color, and he breathed noisily, gasping as if he'd been hit in the stomach. He took two steps back and leaned against a lamppost.

"Is that the bad news? Are you sure; there's nothing else?"

"No, I promise you, that's it. I just wanted to tell you Tiji died."

Gaspard couldn't hold his sobs back any longer and burst into tears.

"I was so frightened, Mommy! I thought you were going to tell me Azylis had died."

It hadn't even occurred to me. But now, standing there speechless in the middle of the sidewalk, my arms hanging limply at my sides while my son's shoulders shuddered, I was suddenly aware of his trauma. Gaspard had already lived through the unimaginable, losing his little sister Thaïs. He knew that Azylis was sick, and he was dreading reliving the loss. I held him tightly and tried to drown his sorrow in my own.

"Don't you worry, my darling. She's fine. For now we don't have any reason to worry, but I understand why you're sad. You're only ten years old, and you've been through very difficult things. Things that are almost too heavy to bear at your age. Please, don't give up."

Gaspard looked up and blew aside a lock of hair in front of his eyes.

"If Azylis dies, I'll be so sad because I thought she was cured. I just can't even imagine how difficult it would be to live without her. But, you know something, Mommy, it wouldn't stop me liking life. Even if Azylis dies, I won't give up hoping."

He used that word on his own initiative; I hadn't prompted him to it, or corrected or extrapolated what he said. Gaspard didn't use the word "hope," but "hoping." I'd always thought that the two were pretty much synonymous and could be substituted for each other to avoid repetition in a sentence without altering the meaning. I now realized that they were not the twins I'd always thought.

"Hope" and "hoping" are two very different concepts. The hope or hopes I'd nurtured consisted of believing in better tomorrows as a way of coping with difficult todays. So my hope rested in the realization of a concrete wish, in a future that would come sooner or later. But this waiting for a better future was mere supposition; that future could easily not be realized and could therefore disappoint me. Now, thinking of Gaspard, if he bases his hopes on Azylis's being cured, and if things don't turn out that way, he'll be profoundly disillusioned. His hopes will be disappointed. The light will go out, and he'll be plunged into the darkness of despair.

Hoping, on the other hand, is like an act of faith, rooted in a certainty: the certainty of what lies at the end of the road, at the summit of the Himalayas. Hoping isn't conditional; it is firm and concrete. I know what the end of my journey will be, whatever trials I meet along the way. I know what I will find, and who I will meet again up there. Enlightened by this hoping, which is so closely associated with trust, I could get on and live in the present on its own terms, with all its sorrows and joys.

There is an expression: "Hope dies; hoping lives on." I think I understand it now, and I disagree with the adage that hope gives life. Hope allows us to hold on, to hold out; but if our hopes prove impossible, they can lead to despair. And despair can destroy us, perhaps not bodily, but mentally. So it's not hope that gives life; it's hoping. Yes, only hoping gives life.

Not far from where I'm sitting, behind a column, the two women are talking more loudly now, no longer worried about disturbing anyone. The church has emptied, and I'm the only person sitting in the nave. Not unusually for a large, thick-walled stone building, the air is cold and damp. I pull my coat tightly around me, blow onto my gloved hands, and bring my feet up onto the horizontal bar of the chair. I put my elbows on my knees and lean forward slightly to rest my head on the crook formed by my upturned palms. As a little girl I used to sit like this, giving free range to my imagination when my mother told me stories. But a different voice is soothing my ears and filling my head right now: my Thaïs's voice. I'd recognize it in an instant. As I did that Christmas night when I was without her for the first time, and I turned my eyes to the firmament and listened minutely to the glorious heavenly chorus of angels until I could make out her singing.

Thaïs's voice no longer has its childish intonation, yet it hasn't adopted the depth of an adult's voice. It's still happy and serene. Thaïs is always with me, but I still miss her; I'll never get used to her absence. It actually hurts physically when all I want to do is hug her but my arms have to close over empty space. I'm trying to acclimatize to this tangible void; I'm learning to live with something missing. I often speak to her, sometimes without even realizing it. I tell her about who I am, what I'm going through, and what I feel. I'm not alone in keeping a connection with Thaïs, each of us in the family and even beyond has built a new relationship with her. Like Gaspard, who, in the early days, gave his sister an unusual mission: he decided that he should stop learning at school, convinced that Thaïs would whisper all the answers to him. He even persuaded his school friends that it would work for them, and in the schoolyard he traded this miracle solution for the Pokemon cards that were his total passion at the time. The whole thing stopped as soon as his teacher looked into it: the collective incidence of low grades put an end to Gaspard's trading. I can just imagine him handing back the cards from the failed deal and muttering between his teeth, "Come on, Thaïs, you really could have helped me. It's easy for you." Since then he hasn't relied on his sister to do his work for him—not that he thinks she's incompetent, but he realizes that this isn't her job. Now he asks her to give him the strength to overcome fears or cope with problems; sometimes all he wants of her is her unobtrusive, reassuring presence. With a mother's curiosity, I've occasionally asked Gaspard whether he speaks to his sister. His reply comes after a moment's consideration: "Yes, I talk to her, but most of the time she's the one speaking to me."

When Thaïs was born, I thanked the heavens for my pretty little girl, who would be my ally for the rest of my life. Now my ally is in heaven.

The wooden door creaks on its hinges, and I turn around to see a young man come in. He's carrying a worn, old-fashioned-looking leather case, and walks smoothly and purposefully, as if he feels at home here. He stops when he's level with the first row of chairs, puts one knee to the floor, and then turns away, but instead of going back outside, he opens a discreet door and disappears from view up a narrow staircase. My hearing soon picks up where he is: the church is suddenly filled with music as the organ's deeper notes are amplified through the vast space. The young organist has come to rehearse the responses for the next Mass, treating me to a delightful recital.

I pick up my purse and leave my seat, with a little nod to the altar. I step between the columns to the side, glance around, and spot the candles flickering a little way further down. I walk carefully along the side aisle, trying not to let my heels click. There's no one to disturb, but I always feel that the hush of churches is sacred. It's so rare to find anywhere quiet these days. I pass the two gossips, still deep in conversation, and we acknowledge each other without a word. The light guides me to the ironwork candle holders. The first of the holders has neat rows where you can put small candles in colored jars. These are the ones my children always choose, to enjoy the colorful display. Just next to it is a more classic structure with evenly spaced spikes to support dozens of candles dripping down over the iron frame. There are hardly any free spaces. I rearrange the layout to make room for my offering, and take out my wallet to check how much change I have—there's enough. I slip the coins one by one into the metal collection box, and the clinking echoes around the nave. I choose tall, narrow candles, making sure that they're good, straight ones, and then I set them onto the holder, keeping one in my hand. I light it from a neighboring candle that has burned almost right down and cup the wick with my hand while I wait for the flame to grow, then I bring it up to each of my other candles to light them before putting the last one on its own spike. Eight small flames dancing in the half-light of the church. I clear my throat and then, standing smiling at my candles and no longer afraid of breaking the silence, I turn my eyes heavenward and sing softly, "Happy Birthday to you, Happy Birthday to you! Happy Birthday, dear Thaïs! Happy Birthday to you!"

THAT WAS AT ONE MINUTE TO THE HOUR. I'VE HARDLY STEPPED outside before my cell phone starts ringing deafeningly. I forgot to put it on silent, and would have been very embarrassed if it had reverberated around the church. In my confusion I pick it up without checking the screen to see who it is.

"Where are you?"

I recognize the voice and smile.

"I'm outside the church. I'll be there in less than five minutes."

"Okay. See you."

I hang up and head off down the main road, this time allowing my gaze to linger on the boutiques. The window displays look fresh and new, shaking off their winter coats and dressing themselves up in beautiful spring colors. Lemon yellow, bright pink, electric blue, acid orange—the fashions this year look set to be sparkling, and I'm delighted. I'm happy it's nearly springtime; I can't wait to see pale buds on the trees, feel the sun's rays warming, and hear the birds singing. Not that I don't like winter, far from it, but at the end of each season I'm always impatient to move on to the next. I feel no nostalgia for the one we leave behind; it's done its time, and I jig excitedly like a child, waiting for the first signs of change. At the end of summer I'm enthused by the onset of autumn, then to see the next winter, before coming back to life in the spring and savoring another summer. I appreciate the characteristics and all the promise of each season. Loïc says that's a sign of my sunny personality, the way I always see the good side of things. Perhaps he's right. I don't know whether I'm particularly optimistic, but I do love life. And I love living it. I never look to see how full the glass is; I don't wonder whether it's half-empty or half-full. That doesn't affect me. I make the most of each mouthful, without thinking how much I've already had and how much there is left to drink. It doesn't matter how you view the contents of the glass; what matters is what you do with it. I remember something John Lennon once said: "When I was five years old, my mother always told me that happiness was the key to life. When I went to school, they asked me what I wanted to be when I grew up. I wrote down 'happy.' They told me I didn't understand the assignment, and I told them they didn't understand life."

I reach the square and have no trouble finding the café on the corner. Alexandra waves to me from inside, and I go in; the place is packed, with hardly any room between the tables. I squeeze my way through, hugging my coat to me and holding up my purse so that it doesn't catch on a glass or a plate. I come across a woman with her teenage daughter heading for the door. The woman catches hold of her daughter and says, "Let the lady through, honey." I smile and thank them, astonished. Am I really respectable enough to be called "the lady"? Yes, the girl was in her teens, and I'm nearly forty. It's not that I have any complexes about my age, but I can't see that I'm getting older—I don't have time.

I join Alexandra, kiss her icy cheeks, and sit down beside her, facing out: I want to enjoy the view of the square.

"I'm sorry I didn't wait for you outside," says Alexandra. "I was freezing."

"Is Marie on her way?"

"Yes, I just spoke to her on the phone. She was just coming out of the Métro."

Perfectly on cue, Marie appears through the door to the café. She waves and cries, "Hi, girls!" from the doorway, then slaloms between the tables, both hands holding her protruding stomach to protect it from potential knocks. When she reaches us, she drops down into a chair, exhausted.

"So many people, in the subway, on the street, in here! I thought I'd never make it. Is something special happening today?"

"At breakfast this morning Gaspard said February 29 should be a holiday. Maybe other people have had the same idea . . ."

The waiter comes over to take our order. True to her Italian roots, Alexandra orders a strong espresso, and I choose a cappuccino. Marie orders cheese on toast with a green salad.

"I never got around to having lunch," she explains. "I just came out of my last scan."

"The last one already?" Alexandra exclaims. "When are you due, then? It feels like only yesterday you told us you were pregnant."

"It may feel like yesterday to you, Alex, but it's been centuries for me! I have less than two months left, phew! And they say my baby's doing really well. How about you, Anne-Dau, how are you feeling? Not finding today too hard?"

"Apart from when I first woke up, I think I'm doing better than I thought I would."

"That's hardly surprising," Marie interrupts me teasingly. "You've always had trouble waking up in the morning, whether or not it's February 29. You're a real sleepyhead in the morning, especially these last few years, but even before that. And don't try arguing; I've known you a long time."

I like Marie's honesty, the way she can have a go at me without actually getting at me. She doesn't treat me like some poor, fragile little thing; when she looks at me, she doesn't just see the woman who's been through terrible ordeals or the bereaved mother; she sees me as I am—a normal woman.

A few weeks before Thaïs died, Marie and another girlfriend came over to see me at home. I was distraught and very low that day, and seeing me in this state, she said, "Okay, come on, tomorrow we're going on a shopping spree!" The other friend nearly choked on her coffee, and when I went out to the kitchen to fetch a cloth, I heard her chiding Marie under her breath: "Are you crazy? What were you thinking? You can't suggest taking her shopping, for goodness' sake. That's the last thing on her mind. She needs to be comforted, not to have her nose rubbed in a lifestyle she no longer has and will never have again." I went back into the living room, saying, "That's a great idea, Marie! It would do me a world of good."

On that occasion, as she still does to this day, Marie dared to act completely naturally. And that's all I need. I know it's not easy for people to work out how to behave around someone who's suffered. I know because I have the same problem. Like anyone else, I come across people in emotional pain, and I stammer before finding the right thing to say, and hover while I try to work out exactly what to do. Very few people will get it right without fail. Most of us are left speechless and paralyzed by other people's distress. One thing's for sure: anything we say is better than an awkward silence, and anything we do is better than keeping an embarrassed distance. Because there is no ordeal worse than engendering loneliness. I have my dear friend Camille as proof of that.

Like me, Camille has lost a child, a beautiful little boy who had an incurable disease. Camille lives on her own and doesn't have much family, but she does have friends, or at least she did before her son died. I called her in the morning on the first anniversary of his death, but she didn't pick up, and I can understand that. I left a message saying that I was crying with her that day and making a point of thinking about him. I didn't say anything more or anything better than that. She called me back that evening, her voice blank and toneless. She described her painful day, thanked me for my message, and then burst into tears as she confided that no one else had been in touch. Her mother and brother had been with her, yes, but not one of her friends had called. Not one. Even though they hadn't forgotten, and I know that: I'd spoken to one of them on the phone the day before, and we'd talked about it.

"I've never needed them more than I did today," Camille said before she hung up, "and I've never felt so alone in my life." I scoured my address book in search of our mutual friends, and left messages with them, telling them to contact her before the end of the day. A little later I received two replies by text a couple of minutes apart. Two identical replies: "I can't. I don't know what to say." And I stood there on my own in my kitchen, shrieking at my unresponsive cell phone, "I don't know what to say, either. But say whatever you want, whatever you can, anything. It's not the words that matter. Have a bit of courage! Do it for her, to save her from drowning."

There are endless dictionaries, how-to guides, and manuals on etiquette, and they will obviously offer you perennial phrases such as "my condolences" and "I'm so very sorry." But nowhere will you find a trace of the ideal wording, readymade and applicable to any painful situation. It doesn't exist. Comforting someone isn't a question of propriety; it's about love. Consolation involves coming out of yourself, not to put yourself in the shoes of the person who's suffering—that isn't possible—but to reach out to her, to go to a place where you can make a connection with her, where her heart opens and her wound closes over.

Whatever gesture you eventually make, you can be sure of one thing: it will be a lifesaver. Like a hand held out to a drowning man, an invitation to stay in this world, reassuring him that he has a place here. Nothing is more isolating than loss or suffering. And nothing more frightening. But the pain is often compounded by another problem, which is sometimes more difficult to bear: loneliness. Mother Teresa understood this fully when she said, "The most terrible poverty is loneliness, and the feeling of being unloved." That's why I avoid any hierarchy of pain, because that implies a distancing effect. At the top of the pyramid, at the furthest point from the base, are those who are deemed to have suffered the most, more isolated than the banished, the plague-stricken, or the untouchable. I can't count the number of times I've had to point out that leukodystrophy isn't contagious, any more than grief itself.

A woman who'd suffered a terrible loss once told me that no one dared invite her to anything since the events that had turned her life upside down; yet that was the one thing she longed for, to get out and have a change of scene to take her mind off things. She'd recently drummed up the courage to say this and to confront her friends' embarrassed silence. They no longer felt that they could speak normally or laugh and have fun when she was around. She'd given up on those friendships and was clinging on, so as to not give up on life itself. "I can just about cope with the grief," she told me, "but not the isolation, not being banished from society."

A while ago there was an advertising slogan in France that went something like this: "Happiness is just a phone call away." Nowadays it's also just a text away, or even an email. Any means of communication is good. When I called Camille's friends back to insist that they do something, one of them said, "But I really can't send her a text, not in a situation like this." But why not? If it's too hard to pick up the phone and make contact directly, why not write a message? Anything's better than silence. As for what you actually say, simplicity is a failsafe option. No one ever tires of being told, "I'm thinking of you," "I'm here if you need me," "Hang in there," or simply "I love you." Because we all need to feel loved.

I want to give a big hug to Marie, Alexandra, and all the others, everyone who was there for us, through thick and thin. I'd like to thank them with all my heart for not giving up, for sticking with us, for still being here today on the painful anniversaries and the happy ones, too. Our friends have been very persevering, and they've never allowed our own behavior to discourage them. I know we haven't made it easy for them, at least we didn't in the early days. Lots of them got in touch when they heard that Thaïs was ill, and after their initial comforting words, most of them immediately asked what they could do to make themselves useful. I can still remember saying, "Can you cure Thaïs? No, sadly not. So I'm afraid you won't be able to help." I hope that people will read more suffering than cynicism into that comment. The only thing that mattered to me then was my little girl's health. Loïc and I wanted to cope with everything else on our own. We felt young and invincible; we felt that it was incumbent on us to take care of Thaïs and manage the situation. We thought that we had to be strong parents, and we even hesitated before employing Thérèse, convinced that having her was a luxury, not a necessity. Nothing happened as we thought it would: we didn't yet know that Azylis was also ill, and we didn't know that we would soon reach our physical and emotional limits. When we ran out of strength and patience, we realized that we'd never get out of this alone. Never. That was when we started calling all the friends who'd offered to help, asking them if they were still prepared to do something. They all said that they were. And we started living again.

This help offered on the one hand and received on the other reinforced our friendships by giving them another, complementary dimension: trust, a trust that allows the receiver to surrender and accept the gift. Loïc and I learned to receive and to ask quite naturally; our friends learned to offer and agree completely openly. Since then we've hardly ever refused help from those dear to us. And this wonderful solidarity has left me with many emotional memories and a few unforgettable anecdotes. Like the one about the pot of mustard.

"HOW COULD I HAVE DONE IT? WHATEVER WAS I THINKING? I'VE really crossed a line this time." I paced up and down the living room, talking to myself out loud, wringing my hands and rubbing my temples. I looked at my watch; it was past eight-thirty. So she'd be here any minute. How was I going to apologize? Would I have the nerve to blame complete exhaustion or a momentary lapse? She was going to hate me, I knew it. How else could she react?

Sophie had called early in the evening when Thérèse had already left but Loïc hadn't yet come home. I'd just finished tending to Thaïs, who was now already sleeping peacefully. Gaspard was lying in bed looking at a book, and Azylis was gurgling in her bed. The house was quiet and settled, and I was just getting ready to make supper when the telephone rang. Sophie's dynamic voice fizzed down the line, and I was happy to hear from her. We talked about everything and nothing, catching up on each other's news, before she asked the fateful question: "Do you need anything?" I looked around, mentally ran over the apartment—no, everything was fine. I was about to tell her this when I remembered that there was something missing, and before I had time to think, I heard myself saying, "Actually, yes, could you bring me a pot of mustard, please? We've run out." She immediately replied, "No problem. I'm on my way; I'll bring one right over," and she hung up. I went back to my cooking in the kitchen, putting off the task of making the vinaigrette until later when I would have some mustard . . . it was only then that I suddenly realized what I'd done.

Sophie doesn't live very close to us. She has children, a family. She too must have been in the middle of cooking a meal or putting children to bed. And there was I like the Queen of England, thinking nothing of asking her to bring me a pot of mustard! Snap my fingers and up they jump! What on Earth had gotten into me? I genuinely did need help most of the time, real help, like taking Gaspard somewhere or watching over Thaïs or Azylis. Right now, though, I had no pressing needs. I was like any other housewife who needed some mustard to make her salad dressing. I could have done without it or called Loïc and asked him to buy some on the way home.

The entry phone buzzed half an hour later. I stammered as I picked it up and heard her call, "Direct delivery from Dijon!" I opened the door to a giant-sized pot of mustard right in my face. Behind the object of my presumptuousness I spied Sophie's radiant smile. And in a flash I understood this enthusiasm of hers: I realized that it didn't bother her that she'd had to go out of her way for a simple pot of mustard. She did it wholeheartedly, in the same way as she would have responded to a real cry for help. What mattered to her was being there, feeling useful, and helping me carry my burden by whatever means. And what I really needed was her friendship—far more than the mustard.

Alexandra and Marie are still laughing as they remember the anecdote. And, as if to justify myself, more than five years after the incident, I add, "But don't worry; I didn't let Sophie go just like that. Loïc arrived soon afterward, and we invited her to stay for supper. We had a really good evening. And the vinaigrette was delicious!"

"Supper's a fair trade for a pot of mustard. In fact, don't forget I'm coming over next Saturday evening if your invitation still stands. Do you need anything? Some mayonnaise or a bottle of olive oil?" Alexandra teases.

I pretend to throw my sugar lumps at her before saying, "I'm really sorry to break up the fun, but I have to go. I have a date. I'm going to pick Gaspard up from school today."

"That's a great idea. He'll be so pleased."

"Well, I hope he will. The other day he told me that when he moves to junior high next year, I can go pick him up if I want to, but if I do, I'll have to wait for him on the corner of the street, not outside the school. So I'm making the most of it before I'm completely *persona non grata*."

We say our good-byes, knowing that we'll see each other again at my apartment on Saturday.

"Extra hot mustard or traditional?" Marie quips as she walks away.

They both burst out laughing. It's good to have friends.

I JUST HAVE TIME TO DIVE INTO THE SUBWAY TRAIN BEFORE THE doors snap shut. It shudders as it sets off, and the wheels squeak on the rails. I sit down on an empty seat and look around me. Most of the passengers are looking downward, deep in their own business. Some have the free papers handed out at the stations, holding them at arm's length and reading them. Others are using their journey as an opportunity to read a book. Lots have earphones in and are listening to music, or are tapping away on their cell phone keypads. Take those two girls sitting side by side, for example, clattering away on their smartphones at great speed and not saying a word to each other. I admire their dexterity; it's like watching a texting competition. I only hope that they're not writing to each other instead of actually talking . . . they both get off at the next station without looking up or taking their thumbs off their miniature keyboards. A sauntering youth comes and sits on the fold-down seat opposite me, and I can hear the clashing notes of the blaring music on his earphones from where I'm sitting. He sees no harm in singing along, perhaps deliberately disrupting the relative quiet. A few people near him sigh pointedly, but no one dares to say anything to him: the Métro is a place of collective individualism.

We come to a stop again, and an elderly lady struggles to get on. No one notices her or at least shows any sign of having seen her. The young "singer" is the only one to get up and say in a deep voice, "Would you like a seat?" The old lady accepts with a smile and teeters over to him. The young man holds the seat down so that it doesn't fold upright while she's trying to sit on it.

"Thank you," she says.

"You're welcome. I'm getting off at the next stop."

"Thank you anyway."

I'd forgotten one of my recent resolutions: not to put too much stock in appearances and, more important, not to be too hasty to judge.

I'm changing lines at the next station myself, and I follow the young man off the train and notice that he turns the sound down on his music when he steps out of the carriage. Maybe it's just his way—a rather provocative way, it has to be said—of combating the general indifference.

As I walk along the platform, I look up at the blue sign standing out against the white tiled wall. It says the name of the station: Pasteur. Up above our heads, on a wide street a few dozen yards from the subway, there is a major children's hospital. One of the best in Paris, in the whole of France even. I was there, within those hundred-year-old walls, six years ago, minus one day. Such memories . . . events that have been revived recently by a very unusual reunion.

My mind goes back to that imposing conference center. I knew that she was there somewhere. I hadn't seen her for years; in fact, I'd met her only once, but her name and face were imprinted on my memory, in the corner reserved for those dark times. That woman had more impact on my life than she could imagine. She was the one who told us that Thaïs had leukodystrophy that fateful March 1. She dropped the bombshell on our happiness, our dreams, and our plans. She was first to witness our unfathomable pain. That doctor came into our lives for a moment, and vanished just as quickly. She was there only for the diagnosis.

For a long time just the thought of that meeting turned my stomach, bringing back the shockwaves of nausea. I thought I'd never see her again, but there was her name on the list of participants for

the colloquium that Loïc and I were attending. And we wanted to
see her.

It was time for a break between two sessions. The audience poured
into the vast reception area, and I rapidly scanned the noisy, compact
crowd, scrutinizing every face. I tried to hone my hearing, wanting to
make out her voice in the hubbub, a voice I'll never forget. Eventually
we spotted her just a few yards away, chatting to a group of people. Loïc
took hold of my elbow and made the first move. We walked toward her
as one; it was just a few paces now. She looked up and peered right at
us, frowning slightly and allowing her eyes to glaze momentarily as she
trawled through her memory. When she focused on us again, her eyes
looked bigger—she'd recognized us.

"Hello, doctor. Could we talk to you for a moment? I don't know if
you remember us. We're—"

"Yes, I remember you well. I know who you are," she interrupted.

She hadn't forgotten. She remembered telling us about Thaïs's diagnosis and the risks to our then-unborn child. She admitted that she'd
asked colleagues for news of our family afterward, so she knew that
Azylis also had the illness, and that Thaïs had died. The obvious tremor
in her voice was not so much a sign of emotion as apprehension. She
felt more comfortable dominating the conversation than letting us
speak, perhaps afraid of what we might say. Perfectly naturally, she
must have thought that we wanted to talk about the day she gave us
the news, that hypersensitive moment. About what she'd said, or what
she hadn't said. About the way she'd broken the news, her tone of voice,
the time she allocated for it. Perhaps she was afraid that we would come
up with the usual criticisms made of doctors in such circumstances,
but we had no desire to venture into that sort of territory. Of course,
there were things we could have gone over, details we could have reex-
amined, but we didn't want to judge that exchange in terms of a good
or bad performance.

A team of professionals had once asked us to evaluate the way we'd
been given the news. We had to say how long it had taken, whether
any aspect of it shocked or upset us, and how we'd felt when we left the
appointment. Ridiculous questions. How long? A couple of seconds or
an eternity, I couldn't tell you; there's no notion of time in situations

like that. What shocked or upset us? Knowing that our daughter was sick and would die, what else?! How we felt? I can't even go there.

I do know that news like this is sometimes very clumsily imparted. People have told me about their own horrifying cases. Incurable diseases revealed hastily with no preamble, between two doorways in a corridor. Dished out by doctors who are offhand, tactless, preoccupied, or in a hurry. This sort of behavior can be explained: the doctor may feel uncomfortable, can't handle his or her own emotions, needs to keep some distance, or is simply afraid. These explanations are no excuse. I remember hearing one doctor say that he wondered whether it was worthwhile taking any special measures when delivering such news, given that whatever anyone did, it was always going to be traumatic for someone to be given a fatal diagnosis. I was floored by such cynicism. Of course news like that is traumatic, and that's exactly why it needs tact, compassion, and humanity. To avoid tipping the scales even further. True, there's nothing to be gained from dragging out the process—the listener soon finds that he or she can't absorb any new information—but he or she will remember the general atmosphere, the context. And this can make it even more of an ordeal, or rather less so.

The moment we were told that Thaïs was ill will always be a terrible memory; that goes without saying. And yet we appreciate that the neurologist had done everything she could to create the right conditions on the day. She took us to a room reserved for us alone, and she asked to have a psychologist present. She spoke in simple but precise terms. She took as much time as was needed but was careful not to let the meeting go on forever or go around in circles. So she gave us the news of Thaïs's illness in the best way possible.

Right now, though, we didn't want to talk to her about the way she'd broken the news to us. She was still looking uncomfortable about talking to us, and I started talking, afraid that she might slip away before we had a chance to say what we wanted to say.

"When we met a few years ago," I said, "you gave us catastrophic news. Nothing was ever the same after that day. We left in tears, terrified of the future, but we were keen to see you today so that we could tell you that we're happy."

We wanted her to know. Because it must be difficult to imagine that a family who's been through something like that could ever taste happiness again. Because she must have pictured us going on living in the state we were when she left us. So, out of loyalty, we felt that we had to tell her that the sun comes out again after the rain: she didn't ruin our whole lives when she told us that Thaïs was ill. She marked them indelibly, but she didn't stop us from living. We hoped that from then on she would remember not only the day she told us the news, but this day, too, even more so. She would have plenty of other difficult diagnoses to announce during the course of her career. Perhaps she would see things differently if she knew that it was possible to recover from that sort of shock. And it was possible to be happy, even though it did take time.

Her shoulders dropped; her jaw relaxed. She sketched the beginnings of a smile. Her apprehension gave way to relief, and she said just two words: "Thank you."

It's not time yet, but there are already lots of people waiting outside the school gates. There's a narrow passageway between the barrier protecting us from the street and the red brick façade of the building, and at the end of every day the place has the same frenetic atmosphere as a trading room on the money markets. The moment the main door opens, people strain on their tiptoes, calling a name and waving their hands. From their vantage point at the top of those few front steps, I don't know how the children make out a familiar face in this crowd. The commotion doesn't last long; in a matter of minutes everyone's left and the street is quiet again.

Gaspard's class always comes out last, so I hang back on the sidewalk opposite and watch the scene. I like this local school. Yes, I know the school yard is too small and so is the canteen, but it's precisely its size that gives this school its human feel. By the end of Gaspard's first year I knew most of the teachers and a good proportion of the families. I've watched the children grow up, their little brothers and sisters be born, the eldest of them moving on. I've formed good, straightforward, solid friendships. By meeting day in, day out on this same sidewalk, often in a hurry, we have something in common. We need only a couple of minutes to exchange our news, divulge some drama, or relate a happy event. Creating a link and maintaining the connection.

The complex dance at the school gates begins with the kindergarten-age children and works its way up through the older classes. I'm chatting with Cécile, Clémentine, and Anne-Sophie, who are also waiting for older children, when a little hand tugs at my sleeve to attract my attention. I turn and see Héloïse's pretty, smiling face, and I crouch down to be on a level with her. Now I can properly see her big green eyes, her nose smothered in freckles, and her chestnut-colored curls.

"Hello, Héloïse. It's great to see you. How are you doing?"

"Hello, Anne-Dauphine. I'm very well, thank you. And how's Azylis?"

"She's very well, too."

"Really?" the child asks earnestly. "Does that mean she's cured?"

Yet again, I realize that my reply could cause confusion. Often when people ask for news of Azylis, they're actually asking how her condition is progressing, while I reply in terms of her current state. I'm not denying that my daughter has a serious illness, but I see it as merely one integral part of who she is. So I reply as I would for Gaspard or Arthur. Today, in completely objective terms, Azylis is well. I'm not referring to her encroaching handicaps and infirmities, but her general state. She doesn't have a cold or the flu or a temperature . . . so she's well.

"No, Héloïse. She's not cured. Azylis can't be cured, you know."

"Yes, I know that. She'll be my fragile friend all her life."

That's what Héloïse calls Azylis. She took a liking to my daughter from seeing her at the school gates, always in her stroller. Having watched her surreptitiously a few times, she came over one day and asked quite openly why Azylis didn't walk and never talked. I was touched by her spontaneity, so I explained that Azylis was ill.

"Either way, you're very pretty," she said, taking Azylis's hand and smiling at her. "And now you're my friend."

Azylis was over the moon.

One day last year Héloïse turned up, excitedly brandishing a pink envelope covered in multicolored glitter. The name Azylis was written in the middle, surrounded by hearts. I was overcome by a wave of emotion before I'd even opened the precious missive: Héloïse was inviting Azylis to her birthday party. As I discreetly wiped my misted eyes,

Héloïse added, "Azylis will be my guest of honor. What sort of games can she play? And what's her favorite cake?"

"I think she'll enjoy pretty much anything. It's the first time she's been invited to a birthday party. Thank you, Héloïse. How old are you going to be?"

"Five, I'm going to be five. That's big, isn't it?"

"Yes, very big. You know, Azylis is going to be five, too, at the end of the month. You're almost twins."

Héloïse looked at Azylis, perplexed, and I could see what she was thinking. Seeing Azylis like this, strapped into her stroller, there was no way of guessing her age. She moved more like a baby just a few months old, but the look in her eye and her smile betrayed a real maturity. Azylis was both so big and so little.

When the great day came, I don't know who was happier—the mother or the daughter. The invitation said to wear a fancy dress, so I didn't waste the opportunity to give a first outing—at last—to the princess outfit Azylis had been given for Christmas. I set her up in front of the mirror in our bedroom for a long time so that she could admire the dress with its full skirt and lovely puffed sleeves in pink satin embroidered with golden thread, the sparkling tiara poised on her prettily arranged hair, and the see-through plastic pumps on her feet, pink, too, obviously. Thérèse, Gaspard, and Arthur all filed past and complimented her on her regal attire. Loïc even called to wish her a happy time.

All the way there I smiled proudly, as if pushing a real princess's carriage. I felt like telling all the passers-by, "We're going to a birthday party." I rang the entry-phone buzzer with the same enthusiasm and announced triumphantly, "It's us!" as if we ruled the world . . . but before the elevator reached us, I'd started shaking. All of a sudden I realized exactly what I'd be confronting in a few minutes' time: a dozen pretty little five-year-old girls running, singing, playing, squealing, jumping, clapping, eating. And in among them my Azylis would be silent and motionless. The contrast pierced me right through the heart. Her outfit suddenly seemed grotesque, and I felt ridiculous, too; I wanted to turn around and go home, take off all this paraphernalia, and get on with my day as if nothing different had happened, brushing aside this momentary madness, this life that wasn't for us. Or at least not for her.

I'd already swiveled the wheels toward the door of the building when a little girl came in with her mother. The child was dressed as a dancer and was clutching the same invitation card as us. When she reached us, she stared at Azylis for a long time before saying, "Oh, you must be Héloïse's friend. What's her name again?"

"Azylis, her name's Azylis."

"Hi, Azylis, I'm so happy to meet you. You have the prettiest dress."

I looked over the hood of the stroller: Azylis was giving her most radiant smile. I realized that she was happy to be here and proud of looking beautiful. Her happiness comforted my dubious heart, and made up my mind for me. The elevator arrived, and all four of us went in.

"Azylis is here!" Héloïse cried when she opened the door to the apartment, and all her guests clustered around Azylis, each of them giving her a heartfelt kiss hello.

My little princess beamed with joy, and before leaving her, I kissed her softly on the cheek and said, "You enjoy yourself and have a good time. I'll be back later."

And I left, feeling so proud. Proud and marveling at my beautiful Azylis, the "fragile friend" who has a gift for conquering hearts with just a smile. And who summons the best in children and adults alike.

"MOMMY, MOMMY!"

Gaspard is calling me from the top of the steps. I wave at him to come over, and he rushes down to join me.

"Mommy, wait; don't go right away. The teacher wants to talk to you."

"Has something happened?" I ask, not expecting this.

"No."

"Are you sure, Gaspard?"

"Yes, Mommy. I promise; I've been very good. Nothing's happened, but she said she wanted to see you."

The teacher waves at me, beckoning. Most of the pupils have already dispersed, but there's a cluster of them left, playing on the sidewalk while their mothers carry on chatting. I suggest that Gaspard join them while I talk to his teacher. He doesn't need any persuading and slips off to be with his friends.

The teacher takes me into the lobby, and the doors close behind us. Everything is quiet. A forgotten glove, a broken pencil, and a few scudding leaves on the floor are the only vestiges of the bustle in here a few moments earlier. Free of all that childish hubbub, the school suddenly feels strangely silent. The only sound is the hurried steps of the last few teachers clicking on the large floor tiles.

"Good afternoon," the teacher almost whispers. "I'm so sorry to keep you, but I wanted a word."

She looks embarrassed and is nervously rubbing the chalk dust ingrained into the creases of her thumb and forefinger. I start to feel worried.

"Is there some problem with Gaspard?"

"No, it's not that; please don't worry. But, you see, in class today, because of the date, I talked to the kids about leap years, and I asked them what was special about a leap year. Gaspard put his hand up and explained, quite rightly, that there was an extra day, February 29. And he added that it was his sister's birthday."

The teacher pauses, sighs, and then goes on: "I told the class that Gaspard was right and said that his sister could only have a real birthday every four years. The kids got kind of fidgety; they wanted to comment on this, and then Gaspard said very calmly, 'It doesn't make any difference. My sister doesn't have birthdays anymore because she's dead.'"

I can now see why the teacher is so uncomfortable.

"I'm terribly sorry," I say, putting a hand on her trembling arm, "I should have talked to you about this, but I was sure you knew about Thaïs."

"Oh, yes, don't worry; I do know. Everyone in school remembers when your little girl died. What breaks my heart is that, without meaning to, I brought the subject up. Gaspard is a brave boy, and I'm upset with myself for bringing back sad memories for him."

"Don't be upset. You haven't brought up anything bad. Thaïs is a part of Gaspard's life. He can talk about her like he did today quite openly, without his emotions running away with him. It would upset him much more if his sister became a taboo subject, something no one dared talk about for fear of hurting him."

Gaspard was in his first year of primary school when Thaïs died. He was new to this school and probably already had a good many friends, like most children his age, but no true confidant. It so happens that not long before Thaïs died, Gaspard's teacher Claire lost her mother, also just before Christmas. When they went back to school in January, they were both dealing with a loss that was still raw. On the first day, the teacher discreetly called Gaspard over and suggested that they make a pact—"a secret just between us two." Those words were enough to enlist my son, and the terms of the agreement were simple: any time the burden of pain became too heavy for either one of them, they should give a little sign to the other. And the other would support them and console them with a look or a gesture that the rest of the class wouldn't even notice. I was touched when, much later, I heard about this pact. Claire taught my son much more than reading and writing that year. She taught him valuable principles and passed on values that would be far more useful to him in his future life. Thanks to her, Gaspard understood that there were other people suffering like him, and that he could comfort them in spite of his own pain. What a wonderful apprenticeship in solidarity, compassion, and consolation.

He also learned that it was okay to be himself in any situation. He didn't have to put on a persona in the outside world; he could be the same Gaspard he was at home. In company, his suffering was due the same respect as his joys. That's very different from what was said in the headmistress's office when I was a child: "Personal problems should be left outside the school gates."

"DID YOU HAVE A GOOD DAY AT SCHOOL?" I ASK GASPARD, WHO IS walking beside me, leaning forward slightly to compensate for his heavy satchel. He is biting hungrily into a chocolate pastry that's still warm, a compulsory tradition on the days when I come to pick him up. He stops, stares at me wide-eyed with amazement, and shrugs.

"Well, it was just school."

I'm worried that Gaspard's aversion to all things academic will never change. We recently met with the headmaster of his new school in preparation for his move there next year. The headmaster asked him a few general questions to gauge his knowledge and personality, then he asked what his favorite subject was. Loïc and I were astonished to hear him reply coolly, "It's grammar, sir." We didn't pick up on it nor comment, and the meeting ended on a positive note. Almost before we'd shut the door, Loïc and I turned to Gaspard and asked, as one, "So, then, grammar's your favorite subject?"

"Of course it isn't! But what did you want me to say? I couldn't exactly say, 'None of them, except maybe sports; the only things I like are recess and lunch time.' He's the headmaster! He likes school; he's chosen to go there every day when he doesn't have to. I had to say something that wouldn't upset him. I don't understand how anyone can ask a child a question like that! I had to think quickly: math was too risky; he might ask me to do a sum. History was out, too; he might quiz me about some event. So, grammar . . .'"

I sneak a greedy look at Gaspard's pastry. He notices and breaks what's left of it into equal halves, handing me the crustier of the two.

"Why did the teacher want to see you?" he asks.

"Nothing serious. She told me about the discussion you had in class about February 29 and Thaïs's birthday. She wanted to make sure it hadn't made you sad."

"No, not at all. I was happy I could tell people it was her birthday. Then in recess Thomas came over and said. 'That's sad; your sister died too soon.'"

Gaspard stops in his tracks, puts down his satchel, straightens his jacket, and looks me right in the eye.

"Mommy, do you think Thaïs died too soon? I don't think so. I think she died at the end of her life, I mean, you know, *her* life."

How does this child keep surprising me like this? I'm constantly amazed by his angle on things. With his spontaneous thoughts and his childlike view of the world, Gaspard encourages me to think things over. He nudges me into reconsidering what I know, changing the way I think. "Thaïs died at the end of her life." Well, that's stating the obvious! But there's nothing stupid about it, oh, no, because if you look at it closely, this comment of Gaspard's has a lot of meaning.

Every part of me—my mind that never stops looking for her, my body that longs for her—everything about me screams that Thaïs died too soon. Too soon for my mother's heart. Too soon to realize the plans, the hopes, the future I wanted for her. Too soon to go to school, go to college, find work, meet someone to love her, bring children into the world, watch them grow. Too soon, much too soon. And yet . . . does life come down to a sum of years or an accumulation of experiences? Is it only of interest if the boxes have been ticked? Thaïs lived three and three-quarters years. That doesn't seem much in an age when life expectancy has never been greater, with many of us expected to live beyond one hundred. I'm painfully conscious of everything she didn't do, didn't know, and didn't see. She left too soon to have a long life, that's for sure, but she did have a life, a great life. In keeping with

Benjamin Disraeli's words, "Life is too short to be little," Thaïs had time to mark our lives profoundly and ineradicably. She had time to be happy, to laugh, and to cry. She had time to be loved, by everyone. She took the time to love, with a love that makes others want to love. She took the time to touch our hearts, to turn our worlds upside down, to fill us with wonder.

So, like Gaspard, I think that Thaïs got right to the end of her life. Her life wasn't meant to go on for eighty years. Just three and three-quarters years. That doesn't make it any less of a complete existence. We're too often inclined to think, or at least to say, that too short a life isn't really a life, and that too long a life is no longer a life. Which makes me wonder: how many years does it take for us to call it "life" and how many decades to stop? Is it really the duration that matters? Life isn't just a period of time that we appreciate and gauge with each candle blown out. Now I turn to Abraham Lincoln, who said, "In the end it's not the years in your life that count. It's the life in your years." And when I think back to Thaïs's just over three years, I can't help but be moved and think, *Only three years, but so much life!*

Two streets away from our road, I look up and scan the façade of the building ahead of us. My eyes come to rest on the third floor. The shutters are open: Monique must be home. She'd been planning to be back before the end of March, and I'd promised to visit her straightaway. Right now, on this particular day, feels right. I'm worried I won't have time later, and that I'll regret it. I can't decide whether to take Gaspard home first and come back.

"Don't worry, Mommy, I'm a big boy. It's okay, we live just around the corner. I can go home on my own."

When I was a little girl in a pretty, peaceful mountain village in the Haute Provence region, my mom had nothing to worry about when letting my big sister and me walk unaccompanied to nursery school at the end of the street. The only instruction we were given was to not go near the road itself, so the two of us walked along the sidewalk holding hands. I also sometimes went on my own. Mommy didn't worry; I wasn't in any danger. But now I'm uneasy the minute Gaspard ever goes out of sight around a street corner. And it's not so much the cars I'm afraid of.

Gaspard is jigging impatiently; he wants to go home all on his own, but what he really wants is to be a big boy and to be seen as one.

So I let him go. I bite my tongue to arrest the litany of advice that pops into my head before he runs off.

I can tell from the way Monique answers the entry phone, from the tears in her voice, that something's not right, really not right. I hurry up the three floors, choosing the stairs rather than the elevator, as if every second matters. When I arrive, breathless, by her door, I leave my finger on the bell for longer than usual, to make Monique open right away. I hear the clunk of the lock and the clink of a key being turned, and Monique appears in the doorway. I struggle to recognize her: her face, hair, posture, clothes—everything about her has fallen apart. And this is someone who never goes out without impeccable hair and makeup, someone who exhales energy and enthusiasm; she's a shadow of her usual self today. Something about her is broken.

She kisses me, and I feel her wet cheeks pressing against mine. I don't say anything but just follow her into the living room. The curtains are almost completely closed, leaving the room in shadow. A single lamp on a round table is doing what it can to light the place despite its dark shade. I go over to a halogen lamp to switch it on, but, with a shake of her head, Monique indicates that she doesn't want me to. I know that feeling, that rejection of light. It's an expression of terrible inner suffering, suffering that darkens the heart and the mind.

"Please, Monique, tell me what's going on. It's your son, isn't it? I thought he was better."

She doesn't say a word, but her whole body is bent over, almost folded in on itself, and this answers for her. In times of great pain the body curls up like this, trying to find the soothing position of a child in its mother's womb. A time when it was safe and comfortable, already alive but still sheltered.

A few weeks earlier, before Christmas, Monique's younger son was in a car crash. He'd just turned thirty-nine, and was happy and fulfilled. He loved life. He was on his way home just before midnight, and did nothing negligent, nothing wrong. He just chanced across a young driver who wasn't confident at the wheel. Monique received a phone call in the early hours. She was already up, waiting for her coffee to finish filtering. It was her son's friend who contacted her, and she was brusque with him before she knew why he was calling. She still remembers what she said, and her words strike her as very inappropriate now: "For goodness' sake, Matthieu, you don't call people at this time in the morning." Then, nothing, a black hole. And these few phrases in a jumble: "Jean . . . car crash . . . hospital . . . head injury . . . life in danger." She turned them over and over in her head like the pieces of a jigsaw puzzle. Her brain refused to understand their meaning. Eventually she started screaming. She picked up her things, packed a bag, closed the shutters, and turned off the heating. Then she left on the spot to catch a train heading east, toward Alsace, to be with her "little boy" as quickly as possible.

She called me on the way there to tell me. Just before hanging up, she realized that she hadn't thought to turn off the coffee machine. "And my cat, I forgot my cat!" I promised that I would take care of things, and went to her apartment. The janitor, a permanently jovial woman, opened the door to me. I took the coffee pot from its stand, and cleaned out the burned on coffee. It took me a few minutes to find the cat, who was curled up asleep on a pillow in an empty bedroom— Jeans, perhaps. I entrusted him to the janitor, who was delighted to have a bit of company.

Jean was in a bad way when he arrived at the hospital, and the doctors were skeptical about how things would go. Monique stayed by his bedside for days on end, looking out for signs of improvement, like a night-watchman paralyzed by the cold, dark night, waiting for the dawn and the promise of the sun's warm rays. Very gradually, Jean's condition improved; his body dealt with the traumas. He left resuscitation and went to intensive care. Reassured, Monique planned to come home to Paris for a few days before the spring. Just long enough to catch her breath, deal with things that needed doing, and see her cat. So the news had stopped there. It all looked reassuring, and her fear had morphed into confidence . . . only to rear up again all the stronger.

I go over to Monique and try to calm her sobs by holding her to me. She wraps her arms around her stomach as she tells me what has happened: Jean slipped back into a coma two weeks ago.

"Just like that, one morning, with no warning signs. The doctors discovered he'd had a cerebral hemorrhage in the night. He'd complained of headaches the day before. I should have listened to him. I should have realized. He came 'round after a few days, but he's no longer there. His eyes are empty, his voice is empty, his head is empty."

Monique isn't looking at me as she talks; she's staring sightlessly at a point on the ground. Her eyes gaze far away, so far that all my well-meaning strength and kindness won't be enough to console her.

"The doctors are very pessimistic. The extent of the damage is colossal. They think Jean will never recover his faculties."

I'd like to reassure her, tell her that the brain's adaptability sometimes produces miracles. I'd like to tell her about all the people with dreadful head injuries who come out okay despite the predictions. I hold my tongue, sensing that those aren't the words she wants to hear today. They're founded on hypothesis, and what Monique wants is certainty. They wouldn't provide the hope that she needs now.

Monique has probably forgotten that I'm here, despite my vice-like arms around her shoulders. She's almost talking to herself.

"My Jean, my little Jean. What sort of life are you going to have? You're not yet forty and your life's ruined. I'm so sorry, my darling; if I'd have known what was in store for you, I wouldn't have brought you into the world."

A searing pain jolts through my heart. No mother should ever have to apologize for giving her child life. I bring one hand under Monique's elbow and slide the other between her shoulder blades, encouraging her to sit down on the sofa. She meekly lets herself be led. I sit beside her and turn sideways so that I can look her in the eye.

"You couldn't know, Monique. We never know what lies in store for our children. Thank goodness! Otherwise none of us would ever have children. And what if we did know? What would you have done if you'd seen Jean's future in a crystal ball?"

"I'd have said no. His life isn't a life at all, you see."

"And what about the first thirty-nine years? All those happy times? You've always said he was a sunny little boy who grew into a cheeky, daring teenager and then a responsible man."

"But that was before. His life doesn't have any meaning now. It's not worth living."

I can sense the full weight of her despair, and I'm sad to see her like this, deprived of light. If only I could find the words . . . I'd like to ask, "What gives life meaning? Is it the job we do, the family we have, the car we drive, the bank account we pay into? And what sort of life is worth living? The life of the great, the strong, the courageous, the intelligent, the lucky? What is it that really matters in life, Monique?"

I'd like to tell her about Flora.

Flora is nineteen; she's beautiful and happy. And yet she can't walk, can't get out of bed, can't move. And hasn't been able to since the day she was born because of a cerebral problem, which most likely happened during her birth but, according to the doctors, was "undetectable." Those same doctors wasted no time in telling Flora's parents that their baby wouldn't survive, and added, "It'll be better that way, for her and for you." But Flora defied all expectations and survived. Through the ensuing months and years, doctors regularly gave their views on her life expectancy, and Flora always disproved them. These regular prognostications stopped the day the little girl's parents turned to the doctors and said, "You can see she wants to live; she keeps defying your predictions, so let's let her live."

When I met Flora, I was struck first by the extent of her infirmity, but then I was bowled over by her personality. Over the course of our conversation, speaking slowly and haltingly, she confided with a smile, "My problem is I can't do much with my days. It's sad not having a goal in life. So I've decided to do everything I can to make people happy. I devote most of my time to it. Everyone who comes to see me, doctors, nurses, my family, visitors from different organizations—I try to make them all happy, with no exceptions. Quite a job, isn't it? But it's a great job." I'd been feeling low ever since I woke up that morning; Flora put a smile back on my face, for a long time. Making people happy, what a wonderful occupation! Don't let anyone ever say that this young girl's life has no right to be. Every single day she gives it the most beautiful meaning possible: happiness. The meaning of life isn't determined by the trials we confront. A life means what we make of it.

Monique is rubbing her eyes with the palms of her hands to dry her tears. A mother whose heart has been broken always cries like a child. She tugs another Kleenex from the packet and shreds it in her nervy fingers.

"I've never known pain like this. But I've been through plenty, my husband leaving, my parents dying, but nothing to compare with what

I'm feeling today. And do you know what's hurting the most? I feel completely powerless to help my baby. I know he's not a child anymore, but he'll always be my baby in my heart. And now, when he needs me more than ever, I can't do anything to help him. It's unbearable. Unbearable. It would have been better if . . ."

Monique doesn't finish her sentence, but her eyes drift off into the middle distance again for a while. I know. I know how that feeling of impotence hurts. I've felt it. But I know something else, too. Something that overrides that powerlessness. It's my secret. One Thaïs told me. I've never told it to anyone, not in detail at least. Because there's an element of darkness in it, the darkness that threatened to engulf my mind and bury all my better feelings. The darkness I had to overcome.

I take a deep breath and exhale it softly, trying to find the strength and the right words. I close my eyes to help me remember, and the memories are right there, instantly, scrolling behind my closed eyelids. As if it were yesterday.

I SHOULD HAVE GUESSED THAT IT WOULD START AGAIN. I'D SENSED IT, so I should have anticipated it, then I wouldn't have been caught out yet again. Why hadn't I at least left the boxes where I could reach them? I rummaged right at the back of the drawer, shouting, "I'm coming, Thaïs. Don't worry; I'll be right there."

In the next room Thaïs's calling had turned into an uninterrupted moan. I finally found what I was looking for. The box was still sealed up. I grabbed it, clutching it in my shaking hands as I almost ran across the corridor to get back to my daughter's bedside as quickly as possible.

I couldn't say how many minutes the fit had been going on. Two, five, ten? I couldn't count; it felt like an eternity. I'd lost all notion of time. As if her pain expanded the seconds. I worked quickly, cursing the box, which didn't want to be opened, frenziedly pulling out the blister pack and popping out a pill. And giving it to Thaïs at last. I prayed that it would work swiftly and release my little princess from her intolerable agony.

I stayed by her side, squeezing her hands and trying to soothe her with words that didn't convince me. "Hold on, Thaïs, it's nearly over. There you are, I've given you the drug. Come on, my pretty one, come on. Hold on. I'm here. Everything's going to be fine." She screamed all the louder, and my heart constricted.

I felt a tight ball rising up from my stomach into my throat, my back broke out into an icy, cold sweat, my brain had lost the plot. It's inhuman to suffer that sort of pain. Inhuman! No one should ever have to go through this, least of all a little girl of two and a half. I couldn't bear seeing Thaïs enduring these paroxysms; they were so violent that they couldn't be quantified on any pain scale. The drugs I'd given her would relieve her, but their latent period was too long. I couldn't take it any longer. It had to stop. I looked over to the box of pills, and, without even thinking, I heard myself say, "Sweetheart, I can see how much this hurts; it's a nightmare. Tell me if you want it to stop. I'll do anything I can to stop the pain, anything. Even if it's forever."

Yes, right then, I was prepared to do anything. Anything rather than leave her to suffer. I needed only a sign from her, a gesture, a word. But Thaïs said nothing.

Not a sound came from her mouth, not a whisper. She looked at me, her face congested by the scream she was holding back between her clenched teeth. She stared at me in deathly silence, encouraging me to look her right in the eye. And then she held my gaze. "It's okay, Mommy. It hurts, but I know it will soon pass. You've done everything you can. I'm screaming in pain, not in despair, but if you can't bear it, if it's too difficult for you seeing me like this, I'll be quiet. I'll protect you, Mommy, so that you don't have to suffer." That is what I read in those big eyes that looked so serene for a moment, while my own were still tormented.

I huddled against her and sobbed openly. It wasn't for Thaïs to protect me from her suffering, to silence her own pain to spare me from mine. She had the right to express what she felt without worrying about hurting me. As I lay next to her, I realized what it was that hurt me so terribly at times like this: my own powerlessness to help her. The feeling of impotence in the face of her pain was unbearable. It was urging me to find an extreme solution because I felt that that, at least, was something I could do for her.

I rested my head on her chest and spoke softly: "I'm sorry, Thaïs; I'm sorry for what I said. Please don't go thinking I can't cope with *you* any more, my darling princess; it's your pain I can't bear." And I sobbed like a baby as I added, "I so wish I could relieve your pain, but I don't know what to do. I'm your mother, and I don't know what to do. I give you drugs, I ask for new treatments for you, but I feel it's not enough. I can see you're still in pain, and it breaks my heart. What can I do to help you, Thaïs?"

She didn't reply in words, but I felt her heartbeat hammering a little harder just under my ear. As if it wanted to attract my attention, as if it wanted to tell me something. I let my own heart dive deep into hers to find the answer, and in a flash everything seemed clear—it was so obvious!

In that regular beat I heard: "Love me, Mommy. That's all I ask of you. That's all I need." Nothing more; she doesn't expect anything else of me. Why didn't I realize that sooner? Medical care heals wounds, but it's love that allows us to forget the pain; it's words of comfort that relieve suffering. Thank you, my little Thaïs, thank you for changing my heart by allowing it to understand that the answer to suffering isn't death; it never will be. The answer to suffering is love.

As the idea grew clear in my mind, the impotence that had dogged me until then slipped away. I wasn't powerless in the face of Thaïs's pain, and I never would be. I could always love her, and love her more. My mind had a glimpse of new horizons, and my heart felt free. I would now counter Thaïs's inhuman pain with a love that knew no barriers, no restraint, no limits.

I'm struggling to drag myself away from these memories, which stir ambivalent feelings. Thaïs's suffering traumatized me, and left its mark on my memory forever. And my heart, my mother's heart, will always remember the extraordinary love we felt in those terrible times. A love that stopped her from exploding into a thousand pieces, but allowed her to expand, and increase her ability to love.

I feel breathless, and my mind is whirling. Monique is sitting in silence. She's put one arm around my shoulders, and she's now the one consoling me. Her sorrow has calmed for now. It will be back, for sure, probably this evening, as the sun goes down. Our strength often flags in the no man's land of nightfall. Right now she wants to call the hospital to find out how Jean is doing. So I leave her, but before the door closes behind me, she says with a sigh, "I'm frightened. I don't know if I'll be able to cope with his life."

"You'll soon see, Monique. Live one day at a time, and don't think about the future too much. All Jean asks of you for now is to love him. With all your heart."

As I walk home, I'm still haunted by our conversation, and I think it over, along with these words from the playwright Corneille: "The strength of love appears in suffering." Only love has the power to inverse the trend. And not only a mother's love. I remember once meeting a retired medical professor, and while he was telling me about his far-off days heading up a pediatric department, he related a crucial point in his career. He'd been called by a team of terrified nurses to the bedside of a little boy tortured by pain. He evaluated the intensity of the pain and prescribed the necessary analgesics. Unfortunately, the pain didn't respond and only grew worse. Faced with the child's constant screams, he'd upped the dose and added stronger medication . . . until he'd exhausted all the options, still with no success. Unable to relieve his young patient's suffering, he was about to walk out, close the door, and escape to the far end of the department, so as to not be confronted with his own powerlessness. He had in fact decided to give up, but then he changed his mind: he turned around, went back to the little boy, took him in his arms, and rocked him. He stayed like that for a long time, until the child relaxed. The staff couldn't believe their eyes, seeing this great professor, who was often distant and authoritarian, this feared and respected head of the department sitting on the edge of a bed, hugging a child and singing softly. His emotion was still palpable years later as he told me the story. And he concluded with tears in his eyes, "When you think there's nothing more you can do, there's still love."

"GASPARD, ARTHUR? AZYLIS, THÉRÈSE, ARE YOU THERE? HELLO-O, is anyone there?"

No one. There doesn't seem to be anyone in the apartment. I call again, my voice bouncing off the walls and echoing around the rooms. I look in the bedrooms, the living room—all empty. I'm surprised: I've just bumped into Marina, Azylis's occupational therapist, in the street; she'd finished her session and had only just left the apartment. So the children were here only moments ago. Thérèse must have taken everyone to play outside before it was too late. If they went out through the garage, I could have missed them. I'm a little disappointed; I wanted to see them. I think about joining them, but I don't know which park they will have gone to. I picture the two boys racing each other on their scooters and twirling around Azylis's stroller, making her laugh. I hope she's wearing enough clothes; she catches cold easily. I can rely on Thérèse's unfailing vigilance; she will have wrapped her up properly. She'll soon warm up speeding down the slide over and over again as she usually does, while Gaspard and Arthur clamber over the climbing frame. All three of my children like playing outside. It would be easier if we had a house with a garden. Soon, I hope! I resisted the idea of moving for a long time, not wanting to leave the apartment where

Thaïs lived. I wasn't ready for that bereavement. But plenty of water has flowed under the bridge, and I can contemplate it more serenely now, for the sake of the whole family.

I look at my watch. It's just after five, which means it's still tea time. That's good news for me: I've always loved this time of day, especially in winter. I take off my coat and gloves, put down my purse, and go into the kitchen. I stand in the doorway, open-mouthed and wide-eyed. The place is uncharacteristically messy: saucepans, salad bowls, wooden spoons, spatulas, and sundry other utensils clutter the work tops. They look as if they've been abandoned and their users have evaporated. I can hear stifled laughter, and I smile but don't move. Then the laughing starts again, more audibly. I take a furtive step toward the table, then crouch down and find that I'm face to face with Gaspard and Arthur, who are giggling uncontrollably. Thérèse and Azylis emerge from their hiding place at the same time.

Gaspard looks thrilled with the effect.

"We tricked you, didn't we?"

"Yes. I was convinced you'd gone to play outside. But what were you doing hiding under the table?"

"We didn't want you to see us."

Dressed in an apron that almost trails on the floor, Arthur confronts me with a sulky expression, his head lowered, his mouth upside down, and his arms crossed.

"You ruined everything, Mommy," he complains. "You weren't supposed to come into the kitchen. We were making a surprise for you."

"Oh, I see. I'm sorry, but I didn't know. What's the surprise?"

"We're making a chocolate cake with Thérèse," Gaspard explains.

"What a great idea! I haven't had tea yet; I'm going to love this."

"No," Arthur retorts, frowning. "It's not for now. It's the dessert for this evening, because it's Thaïs's birthday."

"Okay, I'll wait 'til supper, then. Come on, let's get cooking!"

The children don't need any persuading. Arthur hitches up his apron, climbs onto a chair, and breaks a bar of chocolate into a saucepan. Gaspard weighs the sugar, butter, and flour. He checks the recipe in front of him and gives instructions to his kitchen assistants. Azylis is also part of the team. Comfortably installed in her made-to-measure molded chair on wheels, and with her head steadied by a chinrest, she's beating the egg whites. Thérèse is helping her hold the electric whisk, and Azylis shudders and laughs as the vibrations run up her arm.

The kids give me permission to stay, but I'm instructed not to interfere in the making of the cake. "'Cause it's not a surprise anymore," Arthur says wistfully. So I keep myself to myself, filling the kettle, choosing a warm, fragrant tea, and pouring the bubbling water over the desiccated leaves to watch them dilate. I toast some bread and spread it with salted butter while it's still warm. Then I sit at the table and watch the impressive team busying away in front of me. Thérèse keeps a close eye on the proceedings, and everyone has their own job. Soon the smell of melted chocolate fills the room and gets our taste buds going. Unable to resist the temptation, Arthur surreptitiously dips his finger in the pan. Gaspard sees him and gives him a sharp rebuke. Arthur goes in for a second dip, Gaspard gets angry . . . and an argument is underway. Their cooperation was short-lived, as it often is.

"Come on, boys!" I intervene with a sigh. "Don't argue; you're making a beautiful cake."

"But he started it!" they both reply at the same time, each accusing the other. Their voices get louder as they hurl silly names at each other, and they're off again. Arthur is brandishing a wooden spoon laden with molten chocolate, and Gaspard is dousing him with flour. Thérèse separates them before the kitchen is completely trashed. They both carry on muttering for a while before getting back to what they were doing as if nothing had happened.

Azylis watches the scene in a slightly detached way, apparently not in the least disturbed by her brothers' squabbling. It upsets me seeing my boys quarrelling; I wish they could get on perfectly. Loïc is the eldest of several children, and he frequently tries to reassure me, telling me that there's nothing more normal than scraps between siblings, even quite heated ones. Most of the time I manage to accept this, but I can't help but feel that our very unusual circumstances add extra difficulties to their relationship. There's a big age gap between Gaspard and Arthur, but there is also more than those seven years between them; sadly, there's a lot more than that. In that gap there's an absence, an experience, a story. There are two little sisters with whom Gaspard can neither play nor argue. Of course, he likes spending time with Azylis, and takes a genuine interest in what she does, but that's not the same as having a sturdy brother who would like the same things and play the same games as he does.

Gaspard begged relentlessly for a younger brother, and was feverishly excited all throughout my pregnancy. When Arthur was born, he ran to the maternity ward and stopped abruptly next to the cot with a crestfallen wail: "But he's just a baby! That's not what I asked for. I wanted a brother nearly my age, to play with. I can't do anything with a baby. He's useless." However much we explained that we all start out in life that small, he saw the arrival of a newborn in the family as an administrative error. After a few days, his growing affection got the better of his disappointment. I'm convinced that Gaspard still has traces of that feeling, though. His frustration doesn't foster animosity toward Arthur, but it reveals everything that our older son has had to forego with Thaïs and Azylis. Which is why there's one thing he longs for: his brother to grow up. While I have only one wish: that Arthur should take his time.

The cake is in the oven now. Gaspard checks the temperature and the cooking time, while Arthur stands with his nose pressed to the glass door of the oven. I finish my tea and pick up the crumbs that have fallen onto my plate, dabbing them with my finger. I suggest playing a game with the children once the kitchen is tidy. Gaspard and Arthur exchange a conspiratorial look, and the older of the two speaks for them both.

"Well, Mommy, we'd really like to play with you, but we'd rather watch TV. We've worked hard to make this cake, you know. It would give us a rest."

I think about this. I don't normally like them to watch TV on a school day, but this is a special day . . . so I agree. And they run off into the living room, whooping enthusiastically.

"I'm choosing the DVD," cries Gaspard.

"No, I am."

"No, Arthur, it's always you. It's my turn today."

And off they go with another argument! This time I leave them to sort it out between themselves. They'll end up coming to some agreement.

Azylis is still in the kitchen with Thérèse. She's savoring a spoon covered in the chocolate mixture, which is a difficult exercise for her uncoordinated hands. She doesn't give up, though; she never gives up. She grins at me with her smeared mouth, and I wipe her face with a damp paper towel.

"Will you give me a kiss, Azylis?" I ask her.

She replies with a dazzling smile and opens her mouth wide. I press my cheek to it, and she purses her lips but makes no sound. We stay together like that for a moment; Azylis needs a little time to do things. She understands everything, very well and very quickly, but she executes her movements slowly. The information struggles to get through from her brain to her body. Her limbs take their time to respond. The lesions on her nerve sheaths handicap her ability to move, robbing her of many functions.

I wait meekly, but nothing happens. Azylis sits there motionless, her mouth pursed. She can't manage to give me a kiss. What is a kiss, anyway? It's so easy, obvious, and instinctive, but it's now impossible for my daughter to do. This small step in the progression of her condition is far from insignificant. It proves yet again that the problem is proceeding unchecked. My heart constricts slightly. Not for long, though; it soon calms, because I know what's going to happen. Azylis will try again and again, very patiently, to give me a kiss. She'll push herself to her limits, until she's absolutely sure she can't do it and accepts the fact. Because she always accepts her limitations. Then she'll find another way of showing us that she loves us. I trust her on that. Her ability to adapt is extraordinary.

Azylis hasn't yet given up; I can feel her breath on my cheek. She's concentrating as hard as she can. I move away slightly and cup her face in my hands.

"Don't worry about it, my princess; I felt your kiss, in my heart at least. It doesn't matter if you can't do it. We can do butterfly kisses if you like."

I bring my face up to her cheekbone and flutter my eyelashes to stroke her cheek. She smiles. And so do I.

I head out of the kitchen so that she can go and join her brothers, and as I reach the door, I hear an unhoped-for sound, a "mwah" that resonates around the room and reverberates through my chest. I turn around and look at my princess's face. She did it! I'm proud of her, of her patience, her perseverance, her faith in herself, all her fine qualities.

I go back over to her and hug her, wiping away a tear on her hair. "Thank you, my Azylis, thank you for that kiss. You're amazing."

In moments like this I can't help but think of Jeanne, and the conversation she and I once had. Jeanne is old enough to be my mother, and I meet her at the school gates because she regularly picks up her granddaughters. I like her elegance and gentleness, and I admire her smile. Because I understand all its depth and strength. Jeanne has two daughters around my age: Catherine and her younger sister, Anne-Sophie. I met Anne-Sophie when Gaspard first joined the school; she had a daughter in the same class, and we quickly became friends. She confided in me with their family story when she heard mine. As a baby, Anne-Sophie's older sister, Catherine, had had terrible convulsions. She survived but sustained irreparable brain damage. Catherine is now nearly forty. Of course she's grown, but her neurological abilities are still those of a tiny child, and she relies on others for all her daily needs.

Since I've known this, I've made a point of exchanging a few words with Jeanne when I see her. We never discuss anything very personal, but we ask for news of each other's daughters. The interest we take isn't mere courtesy; it represents a sincere intention and reinforces a silent complicity.

One day when I was waiting for Gaspard to come out of school, I stood a little way away from the gates. I didn't feel like talking to anyone; I was very low, worrying about Azylis and her future. Jeanne was there, too, a little further along the street. I gave her a nod without moving toward her. She replied with a smile. When we left the school, we were both heading in the same direction. As we walked along, talking about everything and anything, I watched Anne-Sophie's daughters running on ahead, followed by Gaspard.

"You're a lucky grandmother," I said. "Your granddaughters are both as pretty and as sweet as each other. Anne-Sophie has done you proud."

"You're right," she said. "They're adorable. And she's given me everything a grandmother could wish for. But Catherine makes me just as happy as she does, you know. I'm very proud of both my daughters."

I stopped in my tracks, as if I'd been struck. Struck right in the heart. I couldn't move or speak. I studied Jeanne, her white hair, the lines creasing her beautiful face, the age spots on her hands. I was looking at an older woman. And that maturity gave her words a whole other dimension. Jeanne had been by Catherine's side for nearly forty years. Forty years of caring for her, carrying her, washing her, feeding her, driving her around, putting her to bed, and getting her up in the morning. I have no trouble imagining the times when she feels discouraged, exhausted, and anxious. And yet, when it came down to it, Jeanne had been indisputably sincere when she expressed all the pride and love she felt for her daughter. I felt like holding her close to thank her for the gift she'd just given me, without even realizing it. Jeanne had just freed me from one of my greatest fears.

Her comment will never stop lighting the path I have to tread. I think of it every time I shudder as I wonder whether I'll be able to be there for Azylis all through her life, despite her infirmities. Whether I will have it in me to be proud of her, as I am now. Whether I'll carry on being amazed by who she is and what she does. In those moments of torment, Jeanne's peaceful voice reassures me. Yes, all that is possible.

I T HASN'T MOVED. IT'S BEEN THERE FOR SEVERAL WEEKS NOW, immutable. It looks at me pointedly every time I come into the bedroom. I can't not see it, stuck onto the front of the shelf above the desk. Its rectangular shape and fluorescent yellow color attract the eye from quite a distance. I chose a very visible Post-it note to be sure that I wouldn't forget. Every day I put off dealing with it, citing whatever invented excuse I could come up with. When I got up this morning, I resolved to deal with it today; it seemed perfectly appropriate. I've put the decision off from one hour to the next. Azylis's kiss has given me the impetus I was missing. It's now or never.

I peel off the little piece of paper. A telephone number is scribbled in black ink in the middle of it. The writing is slightly shaky. It's mine. I've read this sequence of numbers so many times that I know it by heart, but I've never dialed it. I pick up the phone, rub my thumb gently over the squidgy keypad. Hesitating.

On the other end of the line is Azylis's future. This is the number of a specialist institute, the place my daughter may possibly spend her days for the next fifteen years. The place where she will grow and learn and almost certainly feel fulfilled. She needs somewhere like this because she doesn't go to school. When she was getting close to three years old, we couldn't decide whether to register her for nursery school. She could have gone for the first year, perhaps the second, but at such a terrible price. She would have been constantly confronted with her own limitations and difficulties, not only in the classroom but also during recess and in the canteen. The headmistress of the school was very considerate; she was prepared to move mountains for Azylis to go there. But what was the point?

It was a while before I turned that option down. I happily watch Gaspard's progress as he heads swiftly toward his next school; I was moved when I took Arthur to school for the first time. Schooling is reassuring in that it underlines a child's progress. Every new school year makes me a little heavy-hearted as I realize that, yet again, Azylis will have to stay at home this year. I feel as if her life is going on to one side, off the beaten track, far from the traditional route. And that makes me unhappy. Gaspard doesn't see things in the same way; he thinks it's very lucky to not have to go to school. He regularly tells his sister so when he heads off in the morning. Plenty of others agree with him, like Max, a little boy who came to play with Gaspard one Wednesday afternoon. He was six at the time, and it was in the days when Thaïs was living at home, thanks to the Home Care team.

"Could I go see Thaïs?" he asked me almost in a whisper when he arrived. "I'd like to say hi to her, and to say something else, too."

"Of course. Gaspard will go with you if you like. You do know she's sick, don't you?" I checked.

"Yes, I know. Gaspard told me."

"Okay. Go ahead, then."

Max stopped in the doorway, turned to stone.

"I can't go in," he quavered. "I have goose bumps."

"Really? Let's see."

Max pulled up his shirtsleeve.

"Wow, yes!" Gaspard said ecstatically. "You really do have goose bumps. That's weird. Why is that?"

"Well, I'm kind of scared about how I'll feel seeing Thaïs."

"Don't worry; I'm here. She's just a little girl lying on her bed, you know."

The two boys walked into the room, and Max went right up to the bed. He glanced briefly at the blood saturation monitor on Thaïs's finger, and the oxygen tube running under her nose. His apprehension evaporated when he was met with Thaïs's smile.

"Can she hear me?" he asked, taking Thaïs's hand in his.

"Yes, well, in her own way she can."

Max then turned all his attention to her and said, "Hi, Thaïs. You're so comfortable there. You have a pretty bedroom with wonderful pictures over your bed. Did you do them? Okay, no, I'm being dumb, you can't. You know, there's something I wanted to tell you. I don't know if you realize this, but you're just so lucky not to go to school."

It's enough to make you think all boys that age hate school.

The whole question of school didn't arise with Thaïs. She was far too young and far too sick. The situation is different with Azylis. She's getting older and continues to develop her abilities. Even though her condition isn't stable, the parameters haven't been the same since her bone marrow transplant. Azylis is no longer actually ill; she's disabled. Very disabled. Yes, "disability" is the right word to use about her. I don't like saying it. Not like that, anyway. Not that I'm ashamed, far from it, but society looks on disability far less kindly than it does on illness. I've experienced that firsthand more than once. When I tell people that my daughter is sick, I often elicit instinctive compassion. When I tell them that she's disabled, I notice that most people recoil slightly; it's subconscious, instinctive. I don't like it, but I understand it. Most of us are afraid of the unknown, afraid of anything different. We like everything familiar. Infirmity, be it physical or mental, is one of our anxieties. I so wish that I could convert this unfounded fear into understanding. For my daughter, of course, but not only for her. For anyone who suffers for being different, and for us, too, those of us who are well. So that we ourselves don't go through life handicapped by blinders and narrow-mindedness.

The decision not to send Azylis to school was not made easily; how much more painful, then, to decide to enroll her at a specialized institute. I have to admit that I find it reassuring to know that she's at home, within familiar walls, where I can watch over her, help with her care, meet her physical therapist, her psychomotor therapist, her occupational therapist, and everyone else who tends to her. I don't want her to be far away, not her; she's so vulnerable. I can't imagine seeing her go off in the morning and coming back in the evening, and not knowing what she's done during the day. I do leave her with other people, but only people I know and have chosen: Thérèse, of course, but also Amélie, our regular babysitter, members of the family, and a few friends. I can't picture her in the care of people I don't know. I felt the same fear the first day Gaspard went to nursery school, although I comforted myself with the thought that if things didn't go well, he would have told me. But Azylis can't talk.

I'm a naturally anxious mother, and my anxieties are appeased by well-worn routines and being in control of events. I know nothing about the path Azylis must tread; I'm not familiar with that world. I want to keep her with me forever; I don't want her to break away.

So why is there a little voice in my ear and in my heart saying, "Let her live, let her live her life?" I know that voice; I heard it a few years ago now, in Thaïs's bedroom, in the days when I couldn't leave her side for fear that she might need me when I wasn't there, for fear that she might die without me. It was a constant preoccupation, and it upset the balance of the whole family. I didn't have time for anyone else. I stopped sleeping, stopped going out. And I inflicted myself on Thaïs the whole time, without ever wondering whether that was what she wanted. One day the pediatrician who came regularly to assess Thaïs's condition started to worry about mine.

"Let her live a little," she said gently.

Her words shocked and disgusted me.

"How dare you tell me that?" I replied defensively. "By what right? A child needs her mother, especially in these circumstances. Thaïs needs me."

"Yes, she needs you, but she also needs to live her life. She needs to get on with her own life; we all do. She needs to feel that you trust in her."

I then understood what she'd meant. Children can't learn to walk if we always hold them tightly by the hand. I accepted this, even if it broke my heart. I let go. Because no three-year-old girl spends all her time clinging to her mother, however much she loves her. In the same way as no little girl of nearly six wants to spend all her life at home, under her parents' watchful eyes.

Letting go—that should be the definition of the word "mommy." Looking at it objectively, it seems that nothing could be simpler than letting your child go; in reality, it's so very hard. Because a mother has a visceral belief that those she brings into the world belong to her. That their lives depend on hers, like when they were in her womb, where they were warm and, most important, safe. The feeling is all the more acute with a child like Azylis. To be honest, I don't keep her at home for her sake, but for mine. It soothes me. Here, with Thérèse or with me, nothing terrible can happen to her. But Azylis can't stay on the platform watching the train of life go past. She has her own path to tread, an unusual path, perhaps, but it is hers. Her life has a goal and a meaning. My role isn't to be overprotective, but to travel beside her as she wends her way in her own time. And to trust her, so that when the time comes, she too can find a place in life that suits her.

Azylis, I'm letting go of your hand. Even if it makes me cry, even if it hurts, even if I'm scared, I'm letting go of your hand. Because I love you and because I believe in you. I'm not moving away or stepping back; you're the one moving forward. I'm still here, at arm's length, where you can reach me, and my arms will always be wide open to you. Go on, my darling. You go.

I press the ten digits of the telephone number one after the other. On the eighth I dial a five instead of a six. I start from the beginning again. I hear the slow, regular ringing sound. It's ringing; communication is going to be made. I clear my throat and swallow with some difficulty. I go over the sentences in my head, words I've been rehashing for a long time. I make a note on the corner of the Post-it to not forget to say that they were recommended by the staff at the Les Cerisiers Home Care physical education service, who currently care for Azylis. The ringing goes on and on. I wait a little longer. Just when I'm about to give up, I hear someone pick up. I try a shy hello, but the voice at the other end isn't listening to me; it's the answering machine. I've left it too late in the day, and the place is closed. It opens again at nine o'clock in the morning. I hang up, feeling slightly relieved. I'm still holding the piece of fluorescent yellow paper. I look at it closely before crumpling it up into a tight little ball and throwing it accurately into the trash can. I feel better now. I open one of the desk drawers and take out a block of bright pink, heart-shaped Post-its. I tear one off and write the institute's number on it in big digits. This time my writing is assertive; I'm determined. I stick it where its predecessor was, where it's very visible. I smile and then, speaking out loud with plenty of conviction, I say, "Tomorrow."

I<small>T'S DARK OUTSIDE NOW, AND</small> T<small>HÉRÈSE IS LEAVING.</small> H<small>ER DAY WITH</small> us is coming to an end, and she's going home. It's not far away, but it's somewhere else. Sometimes I envy her; I envy her for being able to turn the page every evening, leaving it all to one side until the next day. Yes, sometimes I envy her. Only sometimes, when the situation gets too complicated, when the weight of it is too much to carry, when the fear feels overwhelming. I wish I could get out, tell myself that it's no longer mine to deal with, believe that my real life is waiting for me somewhere else. Sometimes, yes, but not today. It feels right being exactly where I am.

We've just finished a game of Ludo. It's a long time since I've played it, and it proved a perfect compromise for our varied ages. Azylis sat on my lap and joined in by throwing the die for me. With an ally like her, I hoped I might win, but the boys showed no mercy in sending my counters back to the start more than once. I tried various approaches to dissuade them from attacking me.

"Come on, you can't do that. I'm your mommy," I ventured with a sly smile.

Arthur seemed receptive to this argument, but Gaspard didn't show any sign of relenting.

"All's fair in love and war, Mommy," he replied, sending me right back to the beginning.

Arthur won in the end, and now he's running around the whole apartment, squealing for joy as if he's really won some major trophy.

"What's going on here? Is someone slaughtering a pig?" Loïc asks as he comes through the door to the apartment, intrigued by the cries he can hear.

"Arthur won at Ludo," Gaspard says wearily. "He's been hysterical like this for ten minutes now."

Arthur throws himself at his father.

"Daddy, Daddy, I won! It's the first time in my whole life."

"Arthur, it's the first time in your life you've played that game," his brother retorts.

Loïc puts a hand on Gaspard's shoulder, picks Arthur up in his arms, and comes to join me in the living room. I'm just clearing away the counters and the board that Arthur, in his excessive enthusiasm, has scattered all over the room.

Azylis has been quiet and calm up to this point, but she suddenly starts wriggling. Her face lights up: she's seen her daddy. Everyone else ceases to exist when Loïc is around. Right now she's just like any other five-year-old girl turning on the charm for her father, and Loïc melts in the face of her gorgeous smile.

"Hello, my princess. Did you have a good day?"

He doesn't wait for her silent reply, but picks her up in his arms, and she snuggles against him. He takes her to her bedroom to put on her pajamas, while I take Gaspard and Arthur to the bathroom. I run the water and pour in some bubble bath, which forms a thick, fragrant foam. I help Arthur climb into the bath, and Gaspard joins him by jumping over the edge with both feet together.

"Careful you don't slip."

Gaspard doesn't hear my warning; he's already dived into the water and disappears under the bubbles, then resurfaces, blowing like a whale. Arthur imitates this gleefully. I stand in the doorway, making sure that they don't turn the whole room into a swimming pool. I can see Azylis's room from here: Loïc has laid her gently on her bed and is taking a pair of pajamas from the dresser. He's chosen pink ones with matching rickrack at the wrists and ankles.

"Look at your pretty pajamas, Azylis!" he coos. "You're going to look beautiful."

I'm not sure that Loïc is particularly interested in children's clothes, but he knows that his daughter likes to look pretty and laps up his compliments.

I so love the tender way he takes care of her. When he's with Azylis, he develops endless reserves of patience and sensitivity. She's his little princess. And he is indisputably my Prince Charming.

Once, during a consultation about Thaïs's condition, a doctor turned to Loïc and said under his breath, "If you'd chosen any other woman, you wouldn't have had a sick child." It was a logical remark, meant to demonstrate the genetic nature of metachromatic leukodystrophy; it wasn't unkind, but it was still very untactful. Loïc didn't hesitate for a moment and replied, perhaps a little tartly, that he was perfectly well aware of that but that there was only one woman he wanted to have children with, and that was me.

Similarly, if I'd been with a different man I may never have heard of leukodystrophy or any of those other wretched illnesses. Perhaps I wouldn't have been through this sort of ordeal. Perhaps my relationship would have been as untroubled as a stroll across flat terrain, with no mountains and obstacles coming and blocking the view. But then would I have loved as much as I love Loïc? With another man would I have coped with the petty problems of married life, the ones that crop up under the innocent guise of plain weariness, of inevitable routine, of commonplace irritation, or a milestone birthday? I don't know.

One thing I do know is that I didn't choose Loïc for his chromosomes or his star sign. We didn't check our genetic compatibility before falling in love. We were drawn to each other by physical characteristics, by a meeting of minds and a matching of souls. We were seduced by aptitudes, quirks, strengths, and weaknesses, too.

With Loïc, and with him alone, I feel that I can climb these Himalayan heights, even though neither of us was prepared for high-altitude mountaineering. We don't have crampon boots in our shoe closet. We'd never needed them before. We went through life glibly, him in sandals, me in stilettos, convinced that we had an easy path to follow and that our lives would obviously be privileged. The ordeal of our daughters' illness devastated us, but it hasn't annihilated us.

With our without crampons, we decided to climb this mountain, to carry on along our shared path. We undertook this ascent together, taking shaky footsteps, yes, but together. Not side by side, not each in our own time, but roped together. We became dependent on each other, dependent on each other's strengths and weaknesses. Having to encourage and support and wait for each other. To plant each foot in the other's tracks. To reach the summit together. Loïc jokes, saying that during the course of this ordeal he's learned to talk, while I've learned to keep quiet and listen. He's right; we have learned to communicate with each other, but we've also learned to laugh, to cry, to console, to rage, to complain, to tremble, and to hope together. And to love.

Today, battered and bereaved, we can look down over the vertiginously steep mountain path we've climbed. Today we're both standing on top of one of the Everests in our life. Right at the top. In stilettos and sandals.

AZYLIS IS IN HER PRETTY PAJAMAS. I FEEL PROUD; IT'S THE FIRST TIME she's worn them, and I made them. I learned to sew recently; I did it for her. I had such trouble finding clothes that fit her and that would adapt to her circumstances. She needs tops that button up the back, raglan sleeves so that it's easy to put her arms through them, pants with a wide waist to fit her brace but with long, narrow legs. In short, it was a minefield. Anything I found was either too big or too small, so I improvised as a seamstress. I threw myself in on my own at first, but then I had help from Agnès, a friend who's a virtuoso with a sewing machine. Very soon the useful became a pleasure: I love making things for Azylis. And she happily gets involved, choosing fabrics, approving the pattern, watching the work progress. I make unique outfits for a unique little girl.

Azylis is ready for supper and looking lovely. Loïc has even managed to give her two pigtails without her complaining. A father's privilege . . .

The boys are sitting next to each other in the bath, still splashing. Their sister laughs out loud when she sees them: they both have wet hair pulled up into spikes on their head. Arthur has fashioned himself devil's horns and Gaspard a crest like a punk rocker. They have mustaches of foam dripping around their mouths. Who said that children's idea of fun changes with every generation? I used to play like that at their age.

This evening the five of us are having supper together. We thought about inviting some friends, people who were part of "Thaïs's solidarity." The ones who stood in for us, took over from us at our daughter's bedside, and took care of her. The ones who loved her. We'd pictured having a festive dinner to bring this special day to an end, but decided against it. In the end, it didn't seem the right thing to do. What we really wanted was to be just family. Only Thérèse was invited, but she chose to go home. Still, I gave her a slice of cake before she left; she thanked me and said, "Anyway, I'll be with you in my thoughts and prayers."

The children have chosen the menu: homemade spaghetti Bolognese and chocolate cake. No surprises there! I did influence their choice a little to avoid the perennial pasta shells with grated cheese.

Gaspard and Arthur are eating heartily, and even Azylis seems to be hungry for once. Loïc feeds her tiny mouthfuls, making sure that she chews them well so that she doesn't choke. After a while he asks me to take over so that he can do justice to his own plateful before it goes cold. Azylis isn't happy about this. She whines and twists her head as far away from me as she can. I persist, and she only makes more of a fuss, starting to cry to soften up her father. He can't resist, and picks up her spoon again.

Azylis knows exactly what she wants and exactly how to make herself understood. Like all children, she can throw a tantrum or put on a performance. I sometimes get angry, but I have to say that I secretly admire her when she rebels. I like seeing her expressing her own character like this, pointing out that she's not a pushover, and showing us that she understands everything. And, as a mirror image of this, I realize to what extent her usual cheerfulness is a choice. The way she behaves has nothing of the "village idiot" smiling beatifically whatever the situation. She's capable of expressing negative emotions. She has tastes, wants, and wishes, but also dislikes and disapprovals. Which means that when she smiles, when she laughs, she's chosen to. And that gives me so much pleasure.

"Mommy, are we going to put candles on the cake?"

Gaspard wants to bring in the dessert. He's turned the cake out of the mold without breaking it, and put it in the middle of a large round dish. Before serving it up, he's covered it with multicolored chocolate buttons. Yes, it would look pretty with candles, but can we celebrate this birthday just like any other? Is it right to light candles and sing "Happy Birthday"? And who would blow out the little flames now that Thaïs is no longer here? Moments like this are tricky. It's the same when people ask me how many children I have.

The first time I was confronted with this question, I was pregnant with Arthur. It was a plumber who'd come to deal with a leak in the bathroom. As I was seeing him out, Gaspard arrived home from school with Thérèse and Azylis.

"Oh, you already have children," he said. "How many do you have?"

I hesitated before answering. I hesitated because the pain of Thaïs's death was still raw, and I was afraid that I would become emotional in front of this stranger. I also hesitated because I didn't want to make him feel awkward by telling him the truth, to watch his face drop and know that he was thinking, "You idiot, you should have kept your mouth shut. That'll teach you to ask questions when it's none of your business. Poor little woman . . ."

I was about to say, "Three," when I noticed Gaspard waiting anxiously for my reply. He wanted to check what I said, to see whether I counted his sister or she had definitively gone from our family. So I pulled myself together, hoping that the plumber would be satisfied with my answer and wouldn't let his curiosity go any further.

"Four. I have four children."

"Four children! Wow, that must be quite a lot of work. How old are they?"

I wriggled out of that with a flourish: "The oldest is six, and the baby is due at the end of the year."

"Well, you have a beautiful family. Okay, good-bye, ma'am, good-bye, kids."

"Good-bye."

I noticed that Gaspard was thinking of saying something, and I held my breath, but he changed his mind. Almost before the door was closed he turned to me.

"Didn't you want to tell him about Thaïs, Mommy?" he asked.

"No, I'd rather not. If he'd asked where the fourth child was, I would have told him, but I didn't really feel like telling him my life story."

I made a choice that day always to tell the truth, while avoiding going into the details as far as was possible. I don't think there's a right or wrong way to respond in these situations. It all depends on what you can cope with and what you feel like sharing with other people.

We've resolved the question of candles, on which there were various opinions. We put a single candle, a nice big one, in the middle of the beautiful cake the children made. Not to celebrate the eighth birthday Thaïs will never have, but to celebrate her life. Her short, difficult, different life, but the life that was hers. The one she loved, and that we loved.

A candle for a life.

I CAN HEAR MUSIC AND RECOGNIZE THAT LANGUOROUS VIOLIN TUNE. I walk toward it, letting the deep indolent notes of *Méditations de Thaïs* fill my head and my heart. Loïc and I first discovered this opera by Jules Massenet at the time we met, and we were both caught by the spell of this meditation. That's why we gave the name to Thaïs.

Loïc is sitting at the desk, watching the computer screen attentively. It's showing a sequence of photos of Thaïs with this music as a background. I pull up a chair and sit up close to him. I can feel his emotion, and slip my hand into his. His pain as a father bowls me over every time. He would so love to have protected his Princess Thaïs. He would so love to have helped her, to have made her better. One time I heard him whisper, "I'm sorry, Thaïs, I can't save you." He did much more than that. He stayed by his daughter's side right to the end. He tended her, mollycoddled her, and rocked her. He stayed. He was with her, strong yet fragile. He was the best father a little girl could wish for.

Gaspard is in bed reading, and Azylis is half-asleep, clasping her doll in her arms. As for Arthur, I suspect that he's secretly playing with his toy cars under the covers. We sit in silence, leaning against each other like a couple of lovebirds on a branch, soothed by Massenet's meditation and watching the succession of photos appearing at regular intervals on the screen.

"What are you doing?"

Gaspard is standing in the doorway. He got up without a sound, but now we can hear little footsteps behind him. Arthur appears with a car in each hand.

"What's going on?"

"What are you doing here, boys? You should be in bed."

"I heard music, so I came to have a look," Gaspard explains, sitting down between us. "So what are you doing?"

"We're looking at pictures of Thaïs."

"Can we stay with you?" they chorus.

"Okay, if you're quiet and well behaved."

Loïc goes to fetch Azylis so that she's not left on her own, and she looks delighted by this idea of his. He sits back down in his chair and holds her to him, while Arthur climbs onto my lap. The slideshow starts at the beginning again under our watchful gaze. The five of us laugh out loud as we admire Thaïs in fancy dress or with food on her face, looking mischievous or happy. Arthur asks us to tell him the anecdotes, and Gaspard remembers them incredibly clearly. He's the one doing the talking, and we fill in details when they're needed. No one comments when Thaïs looks sick and vulnerable. Those days feel far off now, almost unreal.

The succession of memories ends with a photo of Thaïs taken the day after her second birthday. A beautiful picture of her looking up at the sky, smiling. The meditation on Thaïs gives way to an emotional silence.

Gaspard and Arthur really don't feel like going to bed. They beg to see more photos, more memories. We give in; we too are happy to prolong this special family time. Loïc searches through the computer's memory to rekindle our own. And so we look back over the happy times of our lives, our marriage, the birth of our children, the birthdays, but also those little everyday moments immortalized by the lens of a camera, the moments that, if you put them end to end, make up a life. With every new picture, each one of us makes a comment and dives into his or her own memories. The photos appear in random order, not respecting the chronology of the past. Events overlap, and the years become muddled, giving us a sense of how full our lives are.

"Mommy, what's the most wonderful time in your life?" Gaspard asks, pressing himself a little closer to me.

I have to think. If he'd asked me what was the worst, I would have been able to answer without hesitating. But the most wonderful . . . I think it could be this, this moment, which is nothing exceptional in itself, but it's bringing us together. My moments of greatest happiness are now made of little nothings. Blooming amid the simple pleasures of everyday life. I feel no nostalgia for the past. The most wonderful time in my life is now.

Loïc pauses the slideshow and goes to fetch the remains of the cake and a bottle of fruit juice. The boys greet this initiative enthusiastically: "It's a party!" Now Loïc switches on the stereo and turns up the volume on a catchy tune. The sequence of photos sets off again, but the boys can't sit still anymore. They dance around us, singing at the tops of their voices. Gaspard takes Azylis's hand and invites her to dance with him by swinging their arms from right to left. She shrieks with delight. Then Loïc stands up and spins around, holding her to him tightly. I don't need any encouragement to join them. No one's looking at the photos now: Gaspard has his arms around his father's waist, Arthur is hanging onto his brother's shoulders, and I'm bringing up the rear. And, still holding Azylis firmly in his arms, Loïc leads us around the apartment, dancing all the way. We're completely carried away, and noisy, and together. And happy.

I turn and catch the eye of each of the people around me, savoring the sight of them. Time discreetly suspends its march, each minute tiptoeing past, so as not to disturb the moment. But of course it will end. The children will go to bed, and we'll soon follow, letting the hours of sleep end this day in silence. This moment will pass, but it will leave an enduring, fuzzy feeling in each of us: the feeling of happiness.

Everything is quiet. The children are now fast asleep, Loïc is just finishing with his sports paper, and I'm reading a book beside him. I put my book down, slip out from his arms, and get up from the bed. I walk out of the bedroom, through the darkened apartment, and into the living room. Thaïs's candle diffuses a delicate light, the bright flame dancing. I go over to it and gaze at it in silence.

I hear the wooden floor creak under Loïc's footsteps as he comes over to me. We stay there together for a long time, standing facing that little candle. It's about to strike midnight. I lean forward slightly, and gently blow on the flame. It quivers, wobbles, and goes out without a sound. Flames always die in silence. For a few moments our eyes still hold the memory of that halo of intense light. Along with that light, the day saw its last few seconds. It's now one of our memories. This very special day is actually quite ordinary.

EPILOGUE

My family isn't as I pictured it. Neither is my life. No more than happiness itself. To be honest, nothing is as I thought it would be.

I had some years of insolent happiness, from my happy childhood to my fulfilled life as an adult. Apart from a few snags, there was not a shadow over the picture. And I didn't want any. I wanted to be happy, at all costs. I hoped that I'd been born under a lucky enough star to be spared all through my life. At the time I believed, as many people do, that suffering and happiness were mutually exclusive, irreconcilable. I was convinced that people who experienced real difficulties could, of course, have the occasional moment of happiness, but not real joy. They were deprived of it because their pain, just like poverty, weakness, and illness went hand in hand with unhappiness.

So how is it that I can now claim to be a happy woman? How can I smile despite what I've been through? Some would say that I've lost my head or can't think straight. They needn't worry; I'm fine.

Over the last six years, I've given a new direction to the meaning of my life. I stop waiting for a number of ideal circumstances to be achieved in order to be happy. I've decided to be happy, today, right now. Every day. The pursuit of happiness is no longer my aim in life; it's become a daily choice, which influences how I go about things.

I take inspiration from "Invictus." I love this famous poem by William Ernest Henley, the one Nelson Mandela so cherished, because for twenty-seven years, it gave him a horizon within his prison walls.

> Out of the night that covers me,
> Black as the Pit from pole to pole,
> I thank whatever gods may be
> For my unconquerable soul.
>
> In the fell clutch of circumstance
> I have not winced nor cried aloud.
> Under the bludgeonings of chance
> My head is bloody, but unbowed.
>
> Beyond this place of wrath and tears
> Looms but the Horror of the shade,
> And yet the menace of the years
> Finds, and shall find, me unafraid.
>
> It matters not how strait the gate,
> How charged with punishments the scroll.
> I am the master of my fate:
> I am the captain of my soul.

This poem is more than one hundred years old, and its form—its vocabulary and octosyllabic lines—might seem timeworn today, but the content has lost none of its powerful lucidity. It encourages me to believe that the events we experience don't dispossess us of our lives. Just as a ship's captain doesn't choose what storms whip up the sea and manhandle his vessel. That makes him no less master on board. Standing at the helm, he decides what action to take to save his ship. The same can be said on terra firma. Our trials are imposed on us, and what happens then? When they swoop down on our lives, do they reduce us to dismembered puppets, buffeted helplessly by the ill winds?

For a long time I was tempted to believe that, to think that we had no option but to suffer our lives, to the very end. But I'm not completely convinced that none of us chooses the hardships in our lives, but we can choose how we are going to live them. Or try to live them. Trying every day, frequently stumbling, sometimes losing heart, like the captain doused in water, tumbling along the slipway and narrowly missing going overboard, but who manages to cling to his boat, works doggedly at the helm, and endures the storm, facing up to it until it finally blows over or he has mastered it.

I was happy before, before all these events, but my happiness was fragile, precarious, because it depended on the circumstances of my life. It was closely tied to boxes I had checked, so it was likely to go off course at the least wave. That brand of happiness vanished along with my illusions of an ideal life. A different happiness has taken its place, deep, solid, and lasting. The same happiness that allowed Thaïs, who was powerless and in pain, to be constantly cheerful. So, like her, nothing can now stop me from "loving life and loving it even if . . ."